A terrifically written, touching, open and honest memoir, perfect for those who enjoy humour, exploring human experiences and differences, and aren't too squeamish.

— AJDA VUCICEVIC, PUBLISHING
DIRECTOR, HARPERCOLLINS
PUBLISHERS

A unique perspective and a thoughtful and honest account of a Physician Associate student's' journey, navigating the challenges of PA education and providing insight into the complexities of healthcare and clinical placements. A recommended read for any prospective student contemplating working in the NHS'.

— PROFESSOR JEANNIE WATKINS,
PROGRAMME DIRECTOR FOR THE
MASTERS IN PHYSICIAN ASSOCIATE
STUDIES, SWANSEA

Chloe's story of the journey a physician associate student takes is accurate and entertaining. Outside of the PA profession, few clinicians truly understand the level of knowledge and skills required to successfully complete this incredibly intense course and become a qualified PA. Chloe shares her own personal struggles – both academic and emotional. She has demonstrated the continuity of care PAs can provide by being part of her practice team for many years. Well worth a read!

— KAREN ROBERTS, READER IN
PHYSICIAN ASSOCIATE EDUCATION AT
BRIGHTON AND SUSSEX MEDICAL
SCHOOL

An entertaining, insightful, and refreshingly honest glimpse into the life of a Physician Associate student.

— DR KATHERINE TAYLOR, GENERAL
PRACTITIONER AND CLINICAL LECTURER

Good Practice

Confessions of a physician associate student

Chloe Brathwaite

Faithful Pages Publishing

To the people who fill this world with compassion, kindness and love.

And to our obstacles, which with time, become our stepping stones.

PREFACE

I started to write this book a few years ago, having been inspired by the book *Confessions of a GP by Dr Benjamin Daniels*.

Since that time, and over the course of writing this book, there has been many ups and downs with the physician associate profession, with the last year or so being quite turbulent.

The aim of my book is simply to share my personal journey of becoming a physician associate, with those who may find it interesting, and I hope that you do.

To respect the privacy of friends and colleagues, all names, apart from two names in Chapter 7, have been changed. The two names which remain, have consented to being mentioned.

To respect the privacy of the Hospital Trusts, all

Hospital names have been changed to a colour eg The Blue Hospital. These hospital names are all fictional.

CHAPTER 1

CUTTING EDGE

The room was bright and white, with an atmosphere so tranquil, you could almost hear the drops of blood as, one by one, they hit the smooth vinyl floor. I considered how long it would be before the single drops merged and turned into a puddle, and the puddle into a problem.

Under normal circumstances, I would have busied myself in trying to be as helpful as possible, cleaning up the growing mess, but this was not just any mess. Bodily fluids came with different rules – rules I had not yet learned. There was lots that I had not yet learned.

This was only my first day, after all.

It was not the blood itself that was unsettling. I was used to blood by now. It was more the dynamics of the scene before my eyes that disturbed me ever so slightly. Her, as she lay unconscious on the bed, with spotlights shining down and her blood decorating the floor below. Us, responsible, standing around the bed where she lay, watching, observing. It all reminded me somewhat of the type of film where the victim, helpless, lies in wait for a superhero to swoop in and save them. I had not considered before that sometimes, it is the good guys who leave behind the trail of blood.

From where he stood opposite me on the other side of the bed, the surgeon caught me staring, my eyes fixed on the crimson blood on the floor, my mind lost in reflection. I cared about what he thought of me. It mattered that he considered me up to the task, whether I was or not. It all mattered, everything counted.

'Don't worry about the blood,' he said casually, as if referring to something much less important, before turning back to the crimson canvas of his artistry. 'Sometimes in this job, things get a bit messy. Like life.'

'OK, great,' I replied, sounding calm and relaxed, though inside I was anything but.

She was a middle-aged woman of average height and build, neatly fitting into the surgical hospital bed on which she lay with her eyes closed and her breath soft and rhythmic. The room that we were in was large, despite us only taking up a small area of it, perfectly centred in the middle of the floor. A couple of members of clinical staff hovered around the foot of the patient's bed, head to toe in personal protective equipment (PPE) like us, repositioning medical implements on a silver trolley clean enough to be used as a mirror. There was another clinician at the head of the bed whose only interest was the bleeping machine that the patient was hooked up to, showing various numbers and shapes in different patterns.

I wondered what the patient was dreaming about, and whether people even had dreams under general anaesthetic. Would she be happy with the outcome, feel this procedure had been worth it? Despite wearing a hospital gown tied tightly at the back of her neck, she was covered from beneath her chin all the way down to her feet in a large, disposable green sheet. All apart from her left leg, which was exposed from the groin of her thigh to the tips of her toes.

That reminded me of how I slept on a sweltering summer night, reluctant to surrender the comfort of my duvet, but allowing a single limb to peek out from underneath and experience all the cool air that it could. Although it would not be long before I no longer felt comfortable sacrificing it to the terrors lying in wait in the darkness surrounding my bed, and I would bring it back under the protection of my covers.

Concentrating my mind once more on the here and now, I contemplated how she had come to be here, unconscious and bleeding. There are two main routes into having a surgical procedure: elective surgery, planned between the surgeon and the patient, and emergency surgery, which is self-explanatory. Varicose vein stripping is an example of elective surgery and is as ruthless as it sounds. It was also one of the first procedures that I observed when I started my placement. It was fair to say that I was thrown in at the deep end.

Varicose veins are quite common, typically occurring at the back of the leg when the vein becomes swollen and starts to protrude through the skin. In a healthy leg vein, valves inside it work together to keep the blood circulating around the body and push it back up towards the heart, but sometimes the valves become weakened or damaged, meaning that they are no longer able to operate properly. The blood then pools in the veins, making them swell.

Apart from being unsightly, varicose veins do not generally cause any medical problems. On occasion, however, they can become painful, and can even affect the patient's skin. If pressure stockings do not help manage the symptoms, the only other solution is to remove the problematic vein entirely. Which was what was happening right now, in this patient's case.

I watched as the surgeon made small incisions with a steady hand-held scalpel into the patient's exposed left groin and at different points along her leg. Each careful incision opened the bloody pink flesh with wounds no longer than a couple of centimetres. He then inserted a fine piece of flexible wire into the first incision at the groin, feeding it along the thigh beneath the skin until it reached the last incision below the patient's calf.

Like he was performing a magic trick, he gently removed the entire length of the wire through the lowest incision at the calf, pulling it out of the body. Attached to the wire was the rubbery blue varicose vein.

After being pulled out, the vein was tied off like a shoelace to reduce bleeding, though there still seemed to be a lot of blood everywhere. The once clean forest-green sheet covering the patient had been painted a deep red, making its purpose clear to me now. Whilst covering her, the sheet did not sit flat, but instead created a groove, channelling the blood to run off it like a small river and drip onto the floor.

I had not had any prior surgical experience, not personally. TV programmes and films did not help me quite as much as I had hoped. Most of the information that I had to go on before starting my first day of clinical placements was hearsay from other students.

Not the students from my course as we, overall, had limited, if any, personal experience about each clinical specialty before we arrived. I mean from the other medical students around the university who were always keen to impart advice and wisdom to us. We represented the shiny new profession that the students around the university were still learning about.

Listening to the medical students, I was interested to notice that all clinical specialties seemed to have been awarded unique stereotypes, as if the specialty itself produced certain characteristics and personality traits within its staff. In the communal area outside the library, a couple of keen informants cornered me one day and told me that the doctors who worked in paediatrics were, by nature, soft and gentle people. I hoped that this would be true. Surgeons, on the other hand, tended to be 'quite cold and abrupt' and 'impatient'. I wondered whether this stereotype had come about because of surgeons' unmatched skills in cutting people open. Or had my informants briefly mistaken these medical professionals for *Marvel* supervillains? I was not sure. More concerning, – from my perspective, anyway – was their insistence that surgeons tended to be 'not good with students'.

Surgeons, unlike those in other medical specialties, do not refer to themselves as Dr, but instead as Mr or Ms, a tradition dating back to the 1800s. Around this time, surgeons were not required to have official medical training and could, in essence, just start cutting people open. It was the introduction of the Royal College of Surgeons that deemed it necessary for practitioners to attend medical school before picking up a scalpel.

Thankfully!

The negativity I had heard ahead of starting my clinical placement in general surgery did leave me slightly nervous. However, the team I was placed with at Purple Hospital, a single bus ride from where I lived – could not have been further from the stereotype I had been led to believe. I should have realised that the pieces of 'information' imparted by eager gossips would hold no more truth than Chinese whispers.

My clinical supervisor during my time on my surgical placement was a softly spoken yet confident consultant, extremely friendly with a passion for teaching and demonstrating to his students what life in the department entailed. He was very tall, which meant that for three weeks, I would have to be beady eyed to spot the standing stool placed in each of the operating theatres. After discreetly positioning and stepping onto it, I would get a clear view of what was happening on the operating table, as if I had just had a rapid growth spurt.

I have been told on various mandatory health and safety training days the importance of protecting your back, and surgeons are no exception. The patient's bed would be adjusted to a comfortable eye level for the surgeon, which in my clinical supervisor's case meant raising it significantly. With at least a foot of height difference between us, it was safe to say that our eye levels were not the same, but an intricate surgical procedure could take much longer than anticipated, so it was essential that the surgeon was comfortable from the very start.

So that was where I found myself on my first day in placement, perched on a stool above a growing pool of blood, watching a troublesome vein being removed. When the procedure was complete, the patient's entire leg was tightly bandaged, allowing for pressure to aid healing. And if all went to plan, by the time the bandages were removed and replaced by support stockings the following day, the patient would have varicose veins no more.

At one point during the procedure, the surgeon, with the help of his clinical team, had to raise the patient's left leg as high as his tall shoulders to more easily, access and remove the parts of varicose vein remaining below the skin surface, using a sharp, thin tweezer-type instrument to fish around the open wounds, pulling out fragments of vein one at a time. When he eventually lowered the leg back to the bed, he informed me proudly that he had 'got them all'.

I decided to supress a smile. He reminded me of Ash searching for Pokémon.

Although general surgery as a specialty covers the entire body, most of the procedures that I observed on my clinical placement tended to involve the abdomen. The reason for this is likely that the abdomen contains so many different organs and structures. The appendix the gallbladder, the stomach itself all occasionally require surgical intervention.

I had assumed, however, that during my time in general surgery, I would be seeing a wider variety of intricate procedures. One day, I would be observing complex brain surgery, the next day the heart, but it didn't work that way.

The abdominal wall reminds me of strong brickwork. It helps to keep skin and fat on one side, vital organs on the other side. However, if there is a weakness, the bigger and heavier structures poke through like a tree root through a patch of worn masonry, producing a protrusion. This protrusion is called a hernia.

Hernias can happen at different sites in the abdomen and the groin, and for different reasons. Anything that increases the pressure inside the abdominal wall can cause a hernia, including pregnancy, weightlifting, chronic constipation, even just growing older, as we all do.

A few days into my general surgery placement, I spoke to a patient who had come in for his preoperative assessment, prior to his routine hernia operation the following week. During this assessment, nurses would carry out the necessary physical examinations before his consultation with the surgeon. The patient was a short man in his late 60s, smiley to the point where I wondered whether his cheeks permanently ached.

The preoperative ward was small, with a handful of hospital beds dotted around the periphery of the room, all of which were empty, giving the nurses plenty of room to work. Whilst cheerfully discussing the previous night's episode of *The Great British Bake Off* with the patient, the nurses were doing things like checking his blood pressure, pulse, weight, and height and asking relevant questions about his current lifestyle, all to make sure that he remained fit and well for his upcoming procedure. The patient seemed altogether unfazed by the thought of being cut open by the surgeon's scalpel, his demeanour more that of someone who had popped to a café for a relaxing cup of tea.

Once the nurses had finished documenting their clinical findings onto the clipboards, they then began unclipping and detaching the patient from various pieces of medical equipment as he sat in a chair next to one of the ward's perfectly made-up beds. At this point, I asked him if I might talk to him about the progression of his medical problem – this is called 'taking a history' – whilst he waited for the consultant to arrive. The patient seemed pleased for the opportunity to have a chat and jumped straight into the story of how he had noticed the lump in his stomach, which had continued to grow and grow despite his best efforts to slow it down by keeping his hand firmly pressed on the area for as long as he could throughout the day. When he realised that functioning with only one free hand was much more difficult than seeking professional medical attention beyond the internet forums where his advice had been coming from, he finally made an appointment to see his doctor. The conversation was all very much what I had expected... until it wasn't.

Midway through our chat, the penny dropped. There had been clues, questions such as how long did I typically take for a hernia procedure and how many times had I carried it out, but the defining moment was when he remarked, 'You look so young to be a surgeon.'

Now, many people told me I still looked like an early teen, despite the fact I was by this time 21. But my age wasn't the real issue here; that was the big, clanging misunderstanding going on. The patient was under the impression that he was speaking not to a student physician associate, and a very inexperienced one at that, but to the consultant who would be performing his operation. Upon realising the error, I quickly and earnestly reassured him that I was *not* a surgeon and wouldn't be carrying out his procedure the following week. I would merely be standing on a stool, observing whilst the operation took place, and only if he consented to me doing so.

I did attend the surgery the following week as planned, though it was very strange seeing this chatty, bubbly patient lying unconscious on the bed, no longer smiling, his face neutral, neither happy nor sad, eyes closed in his anaesthetic-induced sleep. The abdominal wall had been neatly cut open at the site where the hernia was and the intestines – looking like links of raw sausages, fresh from the butcher – were visible through the deep incision. A fine metal mesh was put in through the open wound and sewed into the abdominal wall, adding strength where there was previously weakness.

Part of me regretted having talked to this patient during his preoperative assessment. Our laughter at the case of mistaken identity sprang to mind; I recalled his infectious chuckle and the way his warm eyes sparkled with the pleasure of our shared misunderstanding. With every surgical incision, I found myself wincing as if I was somehow betraying him, causing him pain and distress, even though I knew that he was looking forward to the containment of the egg-shaped lump that popped out every time he laughed, sneezed or coughed. It would have been easier to see a faceless, nameless man in such a vulnerable position, rather than someone with whom I had built up such a rapport.

Before the surgeon started to stitch up the patient's

abdomen, two of the team inside the operating theatre, clad head to toe in PPE, began counting pieces of equipment out loud and annotating a piece of A4 paper attached to a clipboard. Nobody seemed perplexed by this, apart from me. Whispering, I asked the consultant why they were doing this, knowing he was eager for me to learn and had reminded me often to ask as many questions as I wanted.

He explained that everything used during the surgical procedure, such as pieces of cotton gauze, sponges, needles, clips, tweezers, forceps, had been itemised beforehand. Now, each item needed to be accounted for before the patient was stitched back up, to make sure that nothing had been left where it shouldn't have been. The last thing the patient needed was to swap a hernia for a surgical scalpel.

I accepted this answer, even though I quietly thought that it seemed a little over the top. When I got home that evening, I decided to see whether the internet could provide me with any more clarity. Was this counting ritual well known and practised by many? Or was it just my surgical team being over cautious?

To my surprise, Google returned countless reports of what is called 'retained foreign objects post procedure', with general surgery having the highest incident rate. Cotton swabs and surgical instruments were the most common offenders, left inside of the patient after their procedure had been completed and their wounds stitched back up. The retained foreign objects often resulted in significant pain and discomfort for the patient, and sometimes injuries, secondary surgery, lawsuits and even death.

Initially, in my naivety, I believed that if a pair of metal forceps had been left inside of me after a procedure, my self-awareness would tell me immediately that something was very wrong. However, after witnessing just how vast and deep the abdominal cavity is, and how many nooks and crannies there are around the organs, I realised that an object could easily be missed by both the patient and the surgeon. Such an avoidable error would be every surgeon's worst nightmare and something that they would do their absolute best to avoid. Counting all the equipment before stitching up the patient suddenly seemed like a small price to pay.

During a procedure, the way in which the medical scalpel cuts through the skin is very different to how I had imagined it would be. I had been expecting to see the surgeon gently glide an excessively sharp knife across the skin, breaking and parting it as beads of blood slowly formed like tiny red balloons being blown up from inside the patient.

My supervisor explained to me that in some parts of the body, the tiny beads of blood quickly turned into a large pool, preventing the surgeon from having a clear view of what and where they were cutting. A scalpel-type instrument where the blade heated up, burning the skin on contact at the same time as making the incision, prevented this problem via a process called cauterisation. The heat would seal the end of the blood vessels, causing a gentle sizzling noise, reducing bleeding and leaving a clearer view for the surgeon and a cleaner wound for the patient.

Cauterisation, unsurprisingly, produces a mild smokey fume. This slowly permeates the air with a faint smell of burning flesh, which is an accurate representation of what is happening. This particular smell, like nothing I had ever experienced before, made me feel a way I had never felt in my life, and it was not a good feeling. The more the smoke rose, the less confident I was that I could stay upright. Fainting was an occupational hazard for students in a surgical theatre, but it was one that I'd assumed I would be immune to.

Despite a heatwave being forecast for a few days to come, the clinical placements were to continue as planned for me and the other physician associate students. We all had to meet a compulsory amount of placement hours, which meant that we were expected to attend in all extremes of weather, hot or cold.

I was observing a complex surgical procedure on the first day of the anticipated heatwave. The already long procedure was made even longer by an unexpected complication, one that my supervisor was confident he would be able to rectify. However, he informed me that I was to take a break whenever I wanted.

The temperature inside the operating theatre felt as though we were in the tropics, but it couldn't be the air that was warm as it was centrally controlled and regulated. No, the furnace was me. My scrubs were made of cotton, but my clogs, apron, face shield were all plastic, my gloves and mask latex. This sweltering combination, with the addition of the white spotlights directly above my head, was making me feel like I was in a pressure cooker. I was constantly rebreathing my own hot, sticky breath and my whole body felt like it was about to overheat and explode. That would have ruined the sterile environment that had been so carefully created.

Having only been standing on my stool for a few minutes, I already felt desperately uncomfortable. The area under my feet seemed to be shrinking, making me overly conscious of my balance so as not to slip off. As soon as the cauterising scalpel touched the skin, as I had expected, fine smokey fumes began to dance up into the air to the low accompaniment of the inevitable sizzling. One of the clinicians stood at the patient's side, holding a silent hand-held vacuum device responsible for trying to suck up the fumes, but some were always able to escape and cloud the air in a fine fog.

The rising temperature of my body, the fumes from the cauterising scalpel, the gradual opening of the unconscious patient's abdomen, the areas of bowel coming into view like a large slimy earthworm – it became all too much for me. I surrendered to my body, quickly stepping off the stool, sitting down on it heavily and putting my head between my legs, allowing all the blood that had drained from my brain to return.

'Can someone please see to Chloe and get her some water?' I heard my consultant supervisor say kindly. Glancing up, I noticed he hadn't taken his eyes off of the open abdomen, into which both his hands were deeply immersed. I guessed he'd witnessed my slow deterioration in his peripheral vision.

One of the theatre staff hurried over to me and took me by the arm, likely worried that my faculties would fail me and I'd hit the floor at any moment. She led me out of the theatre, placing a plastic cup of cold water that I hadn't even noticed her pour into my clammy hands.

The water was like a magic tonic. As soon as the liquid touched my lips, I finished it in one steady draught, feeling more and more like myself with each drop. The clinician had had to remove some of her scrubs upon leaving the theatre, so she looked more like a friendly human and less like an astronaut about to go on a spacewalk. She was young, her obviously long hair tied round and round itself into a bun at the back of her head and a red mark across her nose where the plastic goggles had sat. Seeing fresh beads of sweat forming across her forehead, which she absentmindedly brushed away with the back of her hand, I felt reassured that I wasn't the only one affected by the day's hot weather.

She looked at me with concerned eyes, asking if I wanted to go home. I might have jumped at the opportunity to head off early, particularly on such a warm blue-skied day as today, but my body was challenging me and I accepted the challenge. Changing into my ordinary clothes and going home would have been a sign of defeat; I wanted to show it who was boss. I was about to enter into the medical profession, and whilst by this point, I knew that I had no desire to work in surgery, I refused to feel at the mercy of what my body would allow of me.

I thanked the clinician for her care, allowed her to help me don a fresh gown, apron, gloves and mask, went back into the operating theatre and reclaimed my stool victoriously. The consultant asked me if I was feeling alright, again with eyes not leaving the patient's open abdominal cavity. I thanked him and reassured him that I was fine.

Later that day, the consultant told me a story.

'One summer, Chloe, I had a student shadowing me, just as you are, and he had taken a liking to the stool you always use. Then too, we had a period of very warm weather.

'I was doing a routine procedure. My student was normally chatty, full of questions, but on this day, he was uncharacteristically quiet. Just as I had made the decision to keep my eye on him, he went immensely pale, as if someone had drained the colour from his body, and his eyes became glassy. Before I could put down my surgical equipment or alert one of the team, the student fainted and fell face first into the unconscious patient's open abdomen.'

I waited for the consultant to laugh and tell me that he was joking. Instead, he concluded with, 'So, the moral of the story is, don't be a hero.' His tone was kind and caring, otherwise his words of concern might have sounded like chastisement, and I was never any good at telling the difference.

He went on to reassure me that the student in question had been fine, as was the patient. The student, once conscious, was cleaned up and sent to occupational health for the necessary interventions, and the patient, still fast asleep and unaware of the chaos going on around him, had his abdominal cavity washed out and sterilised to prevent infection from the student's face.

I had no desire to be a hero, so he need not have worried. I was just trying to get through each day, each clinical placement, each exam to qualify for my future career.

I knew what anaesthesia was in general terms, but had never seen it in action until the surgical placement. With local anaesthetic, the patient remains awake, but is unable to feel a specific part of their body. With general anaesthetic, the patient is unconscious, and due to an interruption of the nerve signals, the brain doesn't process any pain either.

The anaesthetist is responsible for administering this process and monitoring the patient throughout the procedure while the surgeon focuses on their own work. At the end of the surgery, the patient is given medication by the anaesthetist to reverse the effects of the general anaesthetic. After being given this medication, the patient is usually wheeled round to the recovery ward, where they are monitored as they wake up.

After shadowing a straightforward procedure that required general anaesthesia, I followed the patient to the recovery ward. She was expected to wake up, having been given the anaesthesia-reversing medication, but this patient remained fast asleep. The anaesthetist checked her medical chart, reviewing her observations and making sure that she had missed nothing. Everything seemed fine. The patient's breathing rate was normal, her pulse and blood pressure healthy, but she wasn't responding to her name being called, a gentle shake of her shoulders. Even a small pinch didn't bring forth so much as a flinch. The patient was still very much alive. Her monitor proved this, but her inert form suggested otherwise.

The anaesthetist stepped away from the patient's bedside to bleep her colleague for advice and support. The colleague appeared at the patient's bedside a short moment later, and along with the anaesthetist made a plan of what they needed to do next to get the patient to wake up. It had now been a considerable amount of time since the medication had been administered with no response from the patient.

As the anaesthetist started to write notes on to the clipboard, the patient's eyelids flickered and slowly opened into a squint. Immediately, she appeared alarmed by all the pairs of eyes staring down at her.

'Is everything OK?' she croaked.

'It is now!' the anaesthetist replied, looking like the weight of the world had been lifted from her shoulders.

One particular midweek afternoon on the surgical ward, I watched with confusion as my supervising consultant used a black marker pen to asterisk a patient's shoulder as they talked about the upcoming procedure that would be happening within the next hour. When we were alone and away from the patient's earshot, I asked the consultant why he did that.

'Have you ever got your right and left side mixed up?' he asked by way of a response.

I almost laughed out loud. Difficulty in telling my left side from my right was one of many quirks that I struggled with each day, expecting to grow out of it, but never managing to do so. But now wasn't the time to recount my life story, not with surgery about to begin, so I replied with a simple and light-hearted 'Sometimes', a casual smile sealing the deal.

The surgeon went on to explain that whilst human error is to be expected, in surgery, it is important to try to eliminate it as much as possible, even if this involves drawing on patients. It isn't just the surgeons who get the side of the body wrong, but also sometimes patients themselves when they're describing their symptoms. As consultations happen face-to-face with the patient sitting opposite the clinician, this creates a mirror-image effect, which doesn't help. The consultant told me about incidents where the wrong side of the body had been opened up, and wrong limbs and organs completely removed, which was a mistake that I could easily see myself making.

My right versus left problem was by no means my only quirk, though. Another was a tendency for my imagination to kick in and my mind to wander. Spending as much time as I did with patients who were unconscious made me feel almost like an intruder in someone else's dream, trespassing on something intimate and private. I often wondered what it felt like to be infused with medication which induced sleep, how patients felt the moment they opened their eyes. I imagined they would be aware of what had happened, but perhaps with patches of missing information.

Interestingly, this was a feeling that I could relate to personally: like something was missing or wasn't quite right. There seemed to be a difference in the way I fitted in to and viewed the world around me. The feeling I had was hard to understand, difficult to explain, but had been present for as long I could remember. It was neither good nor bad, neither curse nor blessing, but it seemed specific to me. I was just waiting for more information so things would make sense.

And one day, a couple of years back, that anticipated revelation had come.

CHAPTER 2

WHITE COAT SYNDROME

'Even though they call these plastic goggles, I'm sure they're made of broken glass. It's the only way to explain the passive aggressive way they cut into the bridge of my nose and the side of my face.' My friend Emma Jane was complaining about an item of PPE as we put on our thick white lab coats and tied up our hair. It was the usual pre-laboratory-experiment routine.

There was a particular place that I preferred to sit for the human bioscience laboratory sessions: the second row, close enough to the front of the class to be as attentive as possible, but on the last chair to the left, slightly out of the lecturer, Edson's gaze. Just in case any questions he asked were directed at whoever was sitting in his eye line. I likely wouldn't know the answer. I never did.

I had been at the University of Northampton for a couple of weeks, after deciding to take a joint honours degree in health studies and human bioscience, and I was enjoying the course so far, mainly the health studies side. This explored things like population health, sociology, nutrition, and these interested me. The human bioscience side of the degree was also of interest, but with the addition of difficulty and stress. It involved a lot of laboratory work, more than I'd expected. With hindsight, I should have realised this would be the case.

The fluorescent strip lights on the high ceiling, the rows of benches, the uncomfortable and unnecessarily high stools that we had to half sit, half perch on, the aroma of chemicals mixed with the faint smell of burning from the last class's experiments with the Bunsen burner – it was all new and exciting, yet every time that I left a laboratory session, my brain felt stressed out and tired, and it was only getting worse. I wondered to myself why things weren't falling into place like I had assumed that they would by now.

At the age of 18, I thought that I knew everything. Everything about myself at least. I was certain that I already had all of the information I needed, and nothing would come along and surprise me.

It wasn't that I had life all figured out, quite the contrary. My A-level grades were so far down the alphabet that they could barely be seen, so were not good enough for me to apply to study medicine as an undergraduate to become a doctor, which was what I had hoped and dreamed. I had considered retaking them, but this plan lasted all of a few seconds before I reminded myself that I had really studied hard and applied myself as well as I could, and it was unlikely that another academic year would magically change my grades.

After receiving my disappointing results, I went to an open day at my local university in Northampton, more for inspiration than anything else, and it worked. My plan B would be to study a health-related undergraduate course, and then apply for postgraduate-entry medicine afterwards.

We were a varied mixture of people on the course, diverse in terms of age, background, experience. Some already had a successful career, but were looking to change paths. Some were parents, some wanted to expand their knowledge, some had only just left sixth form, like me, but we were all freshers together. However, there was one way in which I differed from the others: they all had a natural aptitude for science, and this was demonstrated week after week by their carefree attitude, their laughs and jokes throughout the laboratory session as they produced perfect experimental results.

Each laboratory session began with us being given a set of instructions for the experiment of the day. Laid out step by step was what we needed to collect, what we needed to do and when we needed to do it. My peers would browse the sheet of paper, and then head to various corners of the lab for everything they needed. There were little grey trays available for us to use to carry the pieces of equipment back to our desks, but most people preferred to challenge themselves and see how much they could carry in their arms with the minimal amount of trips.

My classmates' enthusiasm suggested that the instructions were pretty clear and self-explanatory. Yet I always struggled to know exactly what I was doing, even after reading them over and over again.

There was always the opportunity to ask questions before the experiment began, as Edson silently floated around our benches, making himself available to offer us any help we needed. My problem wasn't that I was too shy to ask for help, but that I didn't know how to formulate a single and concise question that summed up the point because I had no idea what I was doing. I tried to reason with myself on numerous occasions that all the information was on the single sheet of A4 paper provided and I just needed to do exactly what it said, step by step. But I still found it complicated and complex. If a sentence contained more than one single instruction, I'd find myself confused, stressed and agitated, fantasising about slipping out of the laboratory unseen and driving back home.

Sometimes, the experiments required us to work in pairs, and I immediately gravitated towards Emma Jane, a pretty, mild-mannered fellow student. She navigated the laboratory with effortless grace, gathering equipment and placing it neatly into the grey tray to bring to the table in a single trip, whilst others scurried back and forth, returning to their benches with laden arms as the grey trays watched on passively. It was clear that Emma Jane was both familiar and comfortable with lab work, before she even told me that she'd achieved an impressive A-level grade in biology and felt it only natural to carry her interest over to her degree. She was the perfect lab partner to have. Funny, confident in her own skills and experience in an environment that to me was completely alien, yet humble at the same time.

I hadn't worked in a laboratory much during my A-level studies, and the lab work I had done throughout secondary education had been extremely basic, so I was happy that Emma Jane and I had started to build a good relationship from the very first lab session. She enjoyed working with me as much as I liked – and often needed – to work with her.

There were the odd occasions, though, when we were required to work individually, which I found to be less than ideal. As first-year students, we weren't expected to be scientific geniuses making ground-breaking discoveries; our only real responsibilities to begin with were to get familiar with the lab, always wear a lab coat and goggles – even if the goggles hurt our noses – and not to poison ourselves by eating food whilst working with dangerous and corrosive substances. Still, working alone on an experiment was something that I found difficult. In the end, I'd usually give up and work with Emma Jane anyhow. She seemed to enjoy the company.

However, I couldn't piggyback off Emma Jane for the three-year duration of the course. I needed to make my difficulties known.

. . .

After a particularly sweat-and-anxiety inducing laboratory session, where the rest of the class, as usual, seemed calm and relaxed as I fought back tears of frustration, I decided to speak to Edson about how I was feeling. I was unable to work out what my issue was, but there certainly was an issue.

I waited behind to talk to Edson as one by one, my classmates filed out of the room, happy to be finished for the day and already planning their evening of socialising or relaxing. At first, Edson didn't notice me and got straight into collecting equipment that some people had abandoned on their desks, despite being asked to ensure that everything was put away.

'Hi, Edson, are you busy? Please can we have a chat?' I mumbled just loud enough for him to hear as I stood in the doorway, ensuring that all of my classmates had truly gone. I made him jump, but he skilfully caught one of the beakers that tried to leap from his arms.

'Yes, of course! Please, pull up a stool. I'll just pop these away.'

He hurried to the back of the room and transferred the glassware into the cupboards there before anything else could startle him and cause the whole lot to crash to the floor. Then he pulled out a stool and sat on the opposite side of the workbench, looking at me, his expression intrigued. I was sure that my reliance on Emma Jane hadn't gone unnoticed, so I assumed he thought that I was going to say I wanted to leave the course.

As we sat down, I decided to get straight to the point.

Fearing I might change my mind altogether about having this delicate conversation, I wasted no time in telling Edson about how I was loving the combination of health studies and human bioscience, but was finding the lab work that came with the latter impossible and stressful, and slowly, slowly, I was starting not to enjoy it so much. In fact, I wasn't enjoying it at all. I told him how the night before a laboratory session, I wouldn't sleep due to worry, and in the morning, I would often try to convince myself that I was too unwell to attend that day, even when I was in full health and perfectly able to drive myself into university.

'Do you think that my difficulty with following the instructions for the experiments is because I didn't take biology at A Level?' I asked after explaining how I was feeling. My intention throughout the conversation had been to remain calm and casual, slightly nonchalant as I poured out my heart to Edson, a man I barely knew, whilst hoping for reassurance that I wasn't losing my mind as I often thought I was. Edson was a great listener and gave me his undivided attention as I part explained, and part vented. He nodded along with an encouraging 'hmm' in all of the right places, his empathetic facial expression demonstrating that he understood my upset and frustration.

But the reassurance wasn't forthcoming. Instead of telling me that things would get better, but it might take some time – the words I was hoping to hear, Edson passed me a piece of paper from a pile on his desk and asked me to have a read through it. The piece of paper contained instructions for the experiment his next group would be doing.

I read the instructions in my head, and then aloud under my breath, pretending to be calm. It felt as though there were hundreds of them simultaneously jumping off the paper and hitting me around the head, all demanding my immediate attention. I used my hand to cover up most of the instructions, only revealing the first part of the first sentence, a much more manageable chunk of information for me to process. It wasn't long, however, before the stress returned. Fully aware of Edson's gaze, I felt hot tears of embarrassment run down my cheeks.

Edson's expression remained understanding and kind. He handed me a soft tissue, then broke the uncomfortable silence with a question that no-one had ever asked me before.

'Have you considered that you may be dyslexic?'

My mind went back to learning to drive only a few months prior. It was an experience that had been as exciting as it was stressful and terrifying for me.

Being born in July meant that I was one of the youngest in my academic year. In turn, this meant being one of the last to reach rites of passage, like learning how to drive. Some of my friends had passed both their theory and practical test before I was even legally allowed to apply for the little green provisional licence. I had listened to friends talk about their driving lessons – the ups and downs, triumphs and near misses – and concluded that I had already learned so much, I was more than ready to start my own lessons.

It didn't take me long to find a driving instructor, as he happened to be my next door neighbour, James. This meant that we were able to fit in lots of lessons in a relatively short space of time. Sometimes if he had a cancellation, he would text me and ask if I fancied going for a spin. My response would always be that I absolutely did, and there was no need to pick me up as I could make my own way to his house. This became a running joke which we maintained over the entire duration of our lessons.

James had been a driving instructor for many years. He was highly experienced, quiet, calm and softly spoken, gentle in his manner even when I had only been moments away from crashing his beloved car.

Driving is very much a 'learning on the job' activity. However, I found the verbal instructions extremely difficult to grasp when the car was parked up and stationary, let alone moving along the road with other cars and people around. The instructions were not hard, and I knew this at the time. They were simple things like 'OK, now speed up to 30mph' or 'Slow down and change down the gears', but it took an awfully long time for me to process them in my head, and then turn them into actions. Sometimes, this processing delay resulted in James having to use the brake on his side to slow the car down as he instructed me to pull over to the left, where we discussed what had gone wrong and why.

But I didn't know why things were going wrong. Why, despite hearing what he'd said, wasn't I always able to carry out the instruction? It must have looked like I was simply ignoring him altogether. Things like mastering clutch control, manoeuvres, unprompted gear changes, I found relatively easy, but ask me to follow an instruction to do any of these things, and it tended to result in a small amount of chaos.

I even took the wrong turn on my practical driving test, causing my examiner to have to re-route the whole journey in his head like a human satnav. Thankfully, I wasn't aware of my error until he told me with a smile that I had passed, why I had received the minor marks, and then handed me my certificate. I asked how I had still passed despite turning left instead of right, and he said it was because I had done it carefully and safely.

It actually surprised me when I learned to drive, discovering how much I struggled with my left and right – something I hadn't realised before I found myself behind the wheel of a moving car. Funnily enough, on the morning of my driving test, I had agonised over whether to write the letters L and R on the backs of the corresponding hands, small enough that only I would be able to see them. Eventually, though, I concluded that this would only result in me becoming fixated on the letters instead of the road ahead of me, likely with disastrous consequences.

. . .

Edson's unexpected question made me think of all the incidents and situations in my life when I seemed to find things so much harder than those around me. As I sat in the laboratory, lost in flashbacks to different times in my life whilst Edson watched me, eagerly awaiting my response, I wasn't sure what to do, say, or feel. Part of me wanted to laugh, part of me wanted to cry, but neither response seemed appropriate. Whilst trying not to do either, I accidentally did an unattractive combination of both. A strange snort-like sound came from my mouth as a single tear trickled down my cheek.

We continued to talk some more about dyslexia and how it can affect people differently, along with the vast amount of support available, particularly through the university. He knew a great deal about the subject matter, to the point where I started to wonder whether he had personal experience, but I didn't wish to pry, nor extend this conversation for any longer than I had to. The tears were still coming. I was desperate to bring our chat to a close at the earliest opportunity.

Edson, almost reading my mind, stood. He reached for the nearby box of tissues and handed it to me whilst pretending to busy himself with his pile of papers, giving me the privacy to wipe and blow everything that I needed to. He then went on to tell me about the university student centre and its various services. Staff there would be able to help me with my concerns, if and when I wanted to discuss things further. I thanked him for his time, patience and kindness, picked up my bag and slowly walked out of the laboratory, contemplating everything that I'd thought I knew.

I decided not to waste any time and walked straight from the laboratory to the student centre, in particular the disability services building. I needed answers. Although Edson had suggested I sit with the conversation we'd had and see how I felt about it tomorrow, that was just too far away. I didn't need to sit with it, I needed to explore it.

The disability service was in a small glass building on the side of the main university. Despite its slightly intimidatingly clinical outward appearance, its interior was cosy, brightly decorated with quirky art and large plants, some resembling small trees. The staff behind the main desk were enthusiastic and very welcoming.

I gave the smiley woman I spoke to, who was wearing eye-catching multicoloured pom-pom earrings, a brief overview of the conversation I had just had with Edson, surprising myself by getting a bit choked up in the process. Introducing herself as Cathy, she was understanding, helping me finish my sentence, judging correctly what I was trying to say and what I was asking for.

Cathy explained that initially, I was to fill out a screening questionnaire to determine the likelihood of dyslexia. A low score meant a low probability of dyslexia, which helped people decide if they wanted to go ahead and arrange a full diagnostic assessment. This wasn't cheap and would be self-funded.

I told her that I wanted to do the questionnaire right away, I didn't want to waste any time. It came on a piece of sea-blue A4 paper, with a purple clipboard to lean on. I found a quiet corner and took my time answering each question, and once I had completed them all, I handed the paper and clipboard back to Cathy. She looked over the answers, writing numbers in the margins which I assumed to be some sort of scoring system.

My results, as I expected, demonstrated a high chance of dyslexia. It was time to arrange a full diagnostic assessment with an educational psychologist.

Over the next couple of days, I focused my time and energy on nothing else but finding an educational psychologist. The one I chose was based in Milton Keynes and worked from home, and I booked an appointment with her for a couple of days later. My parents were keen for me to postpone the appointment for a few days so that one of them could attend with me, as they were unable to get the time off work at such short notice, but I just couldn't wait any longer. I reassured them that I would be fine attending alone.

Following the directions of my Garmin satnav was as difficult as having James, my former driving instructor, sitting in the passenger's seat, but thanks to Milton Keynes having a multitude of roundabouts, it wasn't too difficult to correct my wrong turns. The educational psychologist accepted my apology with good grace when I arrived both late and flustered.

A short middle-aged woman, she led me through to

her study, which surprisingly resembled a small classroom. There were a couple of tables in the middle of the room, facing in the same direction, with two chairs sitting behind each. A smaller desk stood in the corner, surrounded by files and storage units. I assumed that was where she did most of her work. The walls were a calming pastel colour, the large windows, unobstructed by blinds or curtains, overlooking her neatly kept garden with a generously sized pond.

The relaxing atmosphere immediately helped settle my nerves. This wasn't an exam, but an exercise to help me understand myself better. There were no right or wrong answers.

To start off, we had a long informal chat about my childhood, education, difficulties, home life and general concerns. All the while, she scribbled feverishly in a notepad; I clearly had more to say than I had initially expected. After the discussion came an array of weird and wonderful tasks and puzzles that I completed under her watchful eye. She gave nothing away in her facial expression, her warm smile and gentle gaze consistent. I felt like a pampered lab rat, accepting her offer of juice and biscuits as I continued to work on the tasks set out before me. I did the best that I could with each task, still unsure what I was hoping the outcome of the assessment would be.

The following week, I received a heavy A4-sized brown envelope through the post. It contained the full diagnostic report, which was very detailed – too detailed. I flicked through to find the summary on the last page. This was far more understandable. It confirmed Edson's suspicions, which were now also my own.

I had been diagnosed with the specific learning difficulties (SpLDs) dyslexia and dyscalculia.

I had done a lot of reading about SpLDs, even before the diagnosis, aware of my limitations in understanding what I might be told at the end. SpLDs affect the way in which information is processed by an individual. They impact a person's neurology function, but not their intelligence.

Specific learning difficulties or disabilities is an umbrella term covering a range of conditions. Dyslexia, one of the diagnoses under this term, can affect memory, speed of processing information, the time required to process it, organisation and sequencing. It can cause problems with listening or trying to express oneself verbally. Reading, remembering or understanding instructions becomes difficult, as does maintaining focus. Even spoken instructions are challenging for the person with dyslexia, as my experiences illustrated. Dyscalculia, another term under the SpLDs umbrella, causes difficulty in understanding maths concepts.

Visual stress was another diagnosis that I received following a recommendation from the educational psychologist to see a specialist optometrist. I had mentioned during the assessment that one of the things I struggled with when I read words on a page was that the letters seemed to move around, sometimes forcing me to use my finger to track and almost pin down each word in turn. It didn't happen all of the time, nor did it happen with all words, but it did happen, making reading – my favourite hobby – something of a chore. Despite always having my nose in books, I often found myself rereading sentences and paragraphs due to the words wobbling, which meant I hadn't actually taken in any of what I had read.

I had mentioned this in the past to my parents, resulting in various eye test appointments, but my vision was always found to be perfect. After being seen by the specialist optometrist and diagnosed with visual stress, a term that sounded extremely dramatic, I learned that whilst it wasn't actually a symptom of dyslexia, around 50% of people with dyslexia also suffered from this.

Put simply, visual stress affects the way in which the eyes focus on certain letters, words, even typefaces. It can affect people in different ways, including the blurring of letters, moving of words, pieces of words disappearing altogether, and hypersensitivity to glare from a page or overhead lights reflecting on to the page. I had experienced all of these symptoms at least once.

After I'd received the diagnosis, my next task was to work out how to use all the new information to make my life easier than it had been up to this point. I gave a copy of the diagnostic report to the university disability service as the educational psychologist had made some recommendations on how specific changes could support me throughout the rest of my undergraduate course. There were still over two-and-a-half years left to go.

It was unnerving handing the report over as the information within it was all still so new, so raw and so personal. It felt fragile – exactly how I felt, too.

The period of time that followed the diagnosis was a confusing one. I was conflicted in how I should feel. On the one hand, I was relieved. I had written confirmation that I wasn't losing my mind. My struggles and difficulties with seemingly small and insignificant tasks, which I had experienced my whole life, had a reason behind them and were all explainable. Following instructions whilst working in the undergraduate laboratory was difficult for me for a reason. Reading, something I loved, was challenging for a reason.

I thought back to my early avoidance of analogue clocks due to my struggle to tell the time based on the position of the hands on the face, and deciding that digital clocks were the way forward for me. The diagnosis explained why differentiating between my left and right side remained a constantly unsolved riddle; why letters of the alphabet like p, q, d and b seemed to change independently before my eyes; why I needed things explaining to me as 'reading between the lines' didn't work – I saw no line. Often misinterpreting what people said, missing sarcasm, finding it difficult to express myself and my emotions verbally – all of it was for a reason.

I remember once volunteering to read a scripture from the *Book of Revelations* during a church service. When I had finished reading out loud to the congregation and returned to my seat, my brother was in quiet fits of laughter beside me.

'What's your problem?' I asked, annoyed.

'You kept saying breast, not beast. I don't think that there will be any breasts coming out of the land or the sea, do you?' He continued to giggle until he was shushed by Mum.

Growing up and throughout my teenage years, I felt generally misunderstood by those around me, simply due to the way in which I communicated. People found me funny, quick witted, having a dry sense of humour when I was being completely serious, and conversely, they often didn't understand my humour or laugh when I expected them to. Overall, the diagnosis – understanding the symptoms it described and how I related to them – was like someone providing me with the missing pages of my own diary. Suddenly, the story of Chloe made sense, and it was validating.

However, the relief of validation passed, and then my emotions changed. The next stage was a mixture of grief and remorse. I wasn't naïve to the fact that people all over the world received terrible life-changing and life-limiting diagnoses each day, but whilst mine was neither of these, I still felt loss. Questions and thoughts of blame were bouncing around my head. Should my parents have noticed that something was wrong and picked up on my difficulties and differences? Should my nursery, primary or secondary school teachers have realised that I was struggling to keep up with my peers, despite me always being present and attentive in class? Should I have championed myself and been more open and honest in expressing my daily difficulties, despite the worry of embarrassment?

I started to wonder about the alternative path my life could have taken had this disability been identified earlier. What if I had been diagnosed in primary school? Perhaps I would not have had to have the CT scans on my head, even though I found the process fascinating and thoroughly enjoyable, to try to find the cause of my persistent daily headaches, which I now know were due to visual stress. Perhaps if I had known at sixth form, I could have had help, resulting in more impressive A-level results. And if my grades had been better, perhaps I could have gone straight into medical school, as I had always wanted and planned. Instead, I had to study an undergraduate degree before applying to postgraduate-entry medicine, a lengthy way to follow my passion. There were a lot of questions, a lot of what ifs to process.

However, my university workload wouldn't wait for me to come to terms with my bombshell of information. I had to remind myself how strong and resilient I was, and how much I had achieved up to this point. I had done relatively well at primary and secondary school, leaving with 10 A–C grade GCSEs. I just about completed sixth form, albeit with unimpressive grades, but still, I left with something. And I had got into university – yes, it was through Clearing the week before the start of term, but I did it nonetheless. I held a full driving licence at the age of 17 and had a part-time job in my local hospital. I'd achieved this all with no blood, but plenty of sweat and an exceptional amount of tears.

I had a lot to be grateful for.

The support offered at university was better than I had expected it to be, though I didn't know quite what I had expected. I was provided with an academic support worker called Sharon who reminded me of the educational psychologist who had diagnosed me – middle-aged with a similar hairstyle, build and gentle tone of voice, she was also keen on providing me with biscuits.

Sharon's role seemed to be almost to help me catch up with myself. I needed to navigate the obstacles I faced, now that I had identified why I had them. Sharon worked with me weekly so I could learn ways to improve memory recall, reading to retain information, verbal comprehension and other skills essential to university study.

She even helped me discover which stationery worked best for me, so I could process information better and reduce my visual stress. I didn't know that stationery could have such an impact, but apparently it does, particularly in those with dyslexia. The specialist optometrist, through tests and examinations, identified that blue-inked pens helped with my processing of information and recall of what I had written down, and even improved my handwriting. With computer screens, tinting them slightly to have a blue hue helped with my reading and processing.

I thought back to the initial dyslexia questionnaire I had filled out for the student disability service. It had been on blue paper, and I now realised that the colourful document wasn't just a matter of aesthetics. It was likely many students who filled it in found a blue page easier to read.

Sharon helped me learn how best to do class presentations, given my difficulty with reading out loud under pressure. The specialist optometrist made me tinted blue glasses to reduce page glare and stop the words moving around. I was provided with laptop software, including speech recognition, to help me with my written assignments. Most importantly, I was given confidence.

With all the random difficulties I had experienced throughout my life, until very recently without explanation, I had been reluctant to allow myself to fully be me. I had a deep desire to explore and try new things, but I also didn't want to present myself with more opportunities for failure. I was never shy, but I did hold myself back. The diagnoses, clarity and understanding about myself made me feel like I was finally starting to realise who I was, providing a new sense of freedom.

My struggles did not disappear with the formal diagnosis, but the coping mechanisms and different ways of doing things completely changed my outlook. Dyslexia and dyscalculia didn't need to be the stigmatised curse that I had originally believed. They were part of who I was and had always been. I couldn't change it and had no choice but to go with it.

After my final third-year exam, I went to the university library to continue working on my postgraduate application to medical school, as had been the plan. I had worked hard throughout the three years and was on track to graduate with grades that met the entry criteria for the medical courses I was looking at. I had spent a lot of time working on my personal statement over the months and keeping my eye on the courses and any new important information that I needed to be aware of.

On this particular day, whilst I was reviewing courses, a Google search result mentioned a postgraduate medical course that I hadn't heard of before. I clicked the link to find out more, learning that this profession was well established in the USA, though it remained relatively new to the UK and the National Health Service (NHS). Provided I received the results that I was expecting, I would meet the entry criteria to apply. I had also been working part time over the course of my degree in a local hospital ward, meeting another of the requirements for work experience in a healthcare setting. I continued to read and google all I could find about this newfound career path, as the afternoon turned into evening.

I had secretly been wondering over the past few months whether the academic improvements that I had made since the diagnoses would really be enough to carry me through another four years of intensive science- and clinical-based study. Even after completing the medicine degree, would I truly be up to the years and years of foundation training with even more exams?

After spending the next few days reading as much as I could about it, I started my online application to study to become a physician associate.

CHAPTER 3

EXPECTATION DEVIATION

'Let me show you some pictures of the outfits I bought for myself over the weekend, Chloe. I didn't really have anything professional, so decided to use the excuse to go shopping. Here, look.'

My classmate thrust her phone into my face. I wasn't really one for shopping, or for scrutinising other people's selfies, but I dutifully swiped through her pictures of her posing in different outfits, telling her what she clearly wanted to hear.

'Yes, they look great.'

Our clinical placements were starting soon, and everyone was getting more and more excited. I too was looking forward to them, knowing that I definitely learned more effectively with a hands-on approach, but part of me was intimidated by the thought of having real-life patients with real-life problems. Whilst no-one was expecting me to act as a fully qualified clinician quite yet, being as I was a first-year student only a few weeks into my physician associate course, I still wanted to do my best, however good that might be. The clinical placements would also mean having to swap the comfort of my jeans, t-shirts and coloured Converse for more professional attire. This in turn meant that I too needed to go shopping, which I certainly didn't love.

Clinical placements mean a student being placed in a particular healthcare setting to observe and learn alongside those already within the team. As with most medical and healthcare courses, clinical placements are a key part of learning to become a physician associate. For us, they were made up of a mixture of compulsory placements, which we all had to complete, and a selection of optional place-ments where we could choose the specialty based on our own individual interests. These are called electives.

In year one of the course, we spent half a day each week on our first placement, which was in general practice. We were all sent to different practices around the local area, either individually or in pairs, based on availability. I was sent to my general practice placement alone, which I was secretly relieved about. Being the only student there meant that I felt more comfortable taking things at my own pace without the worry of being compared to my peers, who I believed would be much quicker to learn new skills than I.

I had informed the course leader and lecturer about my dyslexia and dyscalculia before the course had even begun, as I decided it would be in my best interest to be transparent and open from the very start. However, I felt less comfortable sharing this openly with my classmates. We were still all getting to know each other, having been complete strangers to one another only a few short weeks ago. I wasn't embarrassed or ashamed, but felt protective of myself. At least for the time being.

The general practice where I was to complete my clinical placement was in a small town five miles away from where I was studying. It reminded me of my hometown: small, quaint and leafy. The practice was in a large, open and modern building with multiple floors. It was bigger than any other general practice building that I had seen before, although I soon learned it was divided down the middle and shared by two separate practices, one using the right-hand side and the other the left. Each side came with its own waiting room, clinical rooms and staff room.

On my first afternoon, after arriving extremely early thanks to my fear of getting lost, I was met by the practice manager, Jordan. Young and friendly, she was extremely excited to welcome the practice's first ever physician associate student on to the team. I was given a tour of the big building with Jordan imparting important information, while I failed to absorb much of it at all. As a result, I would continually be getting myself lost in the building throughout my placement, even sometimes ending up in the midst of the wrong practice team for the first couple of weeks.

Each placement came with a clinical supervisor, our go-to person and first point of contact for any issues that might arise, to ensure that we students were getting as many learning experiences as possible. My supervisor was a positive young general practitioner (GP) called Daniel. Despite appearing young, Daniel spoke with knowledge and authority which his patients seemed to warm to and welcome. I could tell that he was well liked amongst his patients, even perhaps too much, as evidenced by my first ever home visit.

Home visits are commonplace in general practice. Sometimes, they are prearranged between the GP and the patient days or weeks beforehand. Other times, they are urgent and unexpected, with a home-visit request going in as the GP is about to take a bite of their hard-earned lunch.

I was curious to learn how a consultation in the patient's home would differ from one at the surgery. Would the patient-doctor dynamic be different in a home setting, the consultation length longer? Would the GP be offered lunch? I was glad when Daniel asked if I wanted to go along with him so that I could get some answers for myself.

The patient fell into the unexpected home visit category. A middle-aged woman with no significant medical conditions in her notes had called in, requesting an immediate home visit. I was a little surprised, having assumed that home-visit patients, urgent or routine, would all be elderly or frail, preventing them from being able to make the journey into the practice. Daniel explained that this wasn't the case as there weren't set criteria. Any patient who felt too unwell to attend the practice, but was not so seriously afflicted that they had to resort to calling an ambulance to take them to accident and emergency (A&E), was appropriate for a home visit.

Although our patient didn't live very far away, our time constraints before the afternoon clinic began meant that it was more sensible for us to drive than to walk. After leaving the car in the well-kept designated parking outside the modern development where the patient lived, we buzzed our way into the main block of flats, the patient telling us via the intercom that the door to her flat would be open and we could let ourselves in. She then cut the connection before Daniel had a chance to speak.

After climbing the communal stairs to her flat, Daniel stuck his head round the door and called out to inform the patient of his arrival. At this point, he also took the opportunity to ask if she would be happy for his physician associate student to be present during the consultation. She responded in a slightly sharp tone that she had expected him to be alone, but as I had already climbed the stairs, I may as well come in too.

We followed the sound of her voice, walking through the hallway into the living room, which was very dimly lit. Despite it being the middle of the day, the curtains were drawn. There was a small lamp lit in the corner of the room, but the majority of the lighting was coming from the multitude of fragrant candles flickering all around.

The patient was a full-figured woman, with long dark hair, thick and fluttery eyelash extensions and bright-red lipstick. Despite the poor lighting, I could see that she was an attractive woman, and she knew it too. She was lying on her side along the sofa, facing us as we entered the room, wearing a short leopard-print nightgown that barely reached the middle of her thighs, thin shoulder straps battling valiantly to keep everything in place. A matching robe hugged her body down to the ankles, and beside the sofa were heeled mule slippers with fur trim. Between two of her long red fingernails was a freshly lit cigarette.

I wasn't sure what to say or where to look. Even though this was my very first home visit, I was certain that it wasn't an average one. She hadn't offered us a seat and I didn't like to presume to take one – not that there was any space left on the sofa to occupy either of us. Instead, we both continued to stand slightly awkwardly in the doorway.

Finally, Daniel broke the deafening silence. 'So, how can we help you today, Mrs Smith?'

'Mssss,' replied the patient, prolonging the word into a high-pitched whistle. After Daniel had held her gaze for a while, eventually raising an eyebrow slightly as if to prise the words from her mouth, she explained that she had been suffering from a terrible, terrible cough. Daniel asked more specific questions, taking a history and helping to narrow down on the diagnosis before examining the patient's chest with his stethoscope. At this point, she closed her eyes blissfully.

After Daniel had collected all the information he needed, he told the patient that she was likely suffering from a viral cough that would clear up by itself over the next few days. Far from being reassured, she seemed disappointed with this news.

As we said goodbye and started towards the door, she spoke sharply. 'So, is that it?' she demanded. After some more reassurance, Daniel repeated the self-management advice that he had given her to help her look after herself and feel more comfortable, including cutting out the cigarettes. Then, before she could speak again, we left.

The short car ride back to the practice was a quiet one. I had so many questions about what had just happened, and none of them were clinical based.

'Are all home visits like that?' I blurted out finally.

'Oh no, they most definitely are not!' Daniel seemed perplexed, his facial expression matching my own silent thoughts. 'I'm so glad that you were there, Chloe. I'm not sure what would have happened if you hadn't been acting as my chaperone.'

'No problem at all,' I responded with an air of importance, guessing what my role as chaperone had entailed and, more importantly, prevented.

After a debrief at the surgery, Daniel explained that the same patient had a history of... let's say, inappropriate behaviour towards him. As a result, the team decided that it would be better for the patient to be seen by a female GP in future. And she would be encouraged to attend her appointments at the surgery in person, like everyone else.

. . .

This patient's apparent disappointment at the outcome of our home visit consultation was to become a pattern over the course of my general practice placement. Not so much the disappointment itself, but the expectations of the patient differing from what I assumed, as well as what the GP diagnosed. For example, I'd assumed that the provocatively dressed woman would have been overjoyed that her symptoms indicated an ailment no more serious than a common cold. Instead, she seemed to want the outcome to be more serious, and I wasn't at all used to that concept. Why would anyone want to be told they're *more* ill than they actually are?

Our university lectures were divided up into academic medicine and communication skills, which we called comms. Our comms lectures taught us how best to take a clinical history from patients, asking specific questions in the most appropriate way to narrow down and rule out diagnoses. Importantly, comms prepared us to get the most out of our clinical placements, and then our careers.

One of the common themes of our comms lectures was the acronym ICE, standing for ideas, concerns and expectations. The first point is related to a patient's ideas about their underlying problem when they seek medical advice, which often differ quite drastically from those of the consulting clinician. For example, the agonising back pain a patient describes as requiring immediate emergency surgery may well be resolved simply by the clinician encouraging them to adjust their workstation, making sure that their desk is the right height, the chair supportive.

Similarly, a patient's concerns can be very different from those of the doctor. I remember speaking to an 18-year-old patient during the general practice placement who was complaining of pain following a piercing of her earlobe. A quick examination revealed that her left earlobe was red, hot to touch and very swollen with yellow crusting around her silver ear stud. My own concern was to treat the apparently infected earlobe before it got worse than it already was. The patient's concern was whether she would need to remove the stud, causing her freshly pierced hole to close entirely, meaning it would have been a waste of money. She was at pains – literally – to avoid this at all costs, including an ear infection.

However, during my comms lessons, I'd learned that the patient's concerns, despite differing from my own, are still important because they are important to that patient. It is essential for a clinician to understand this, and also to voice to the patient that we understand their concerns. I did this with the young woman, even as I sought to explain to her that retaining ownership of her right earlobe was more of a concern than the piercing inside it. Eventually, we agreed to try an antibiotic treatment first, and if there was no improvement at our scheduled review, the piercing would need to be removed.

Expectations are about trying to determine what it is that the patient actually wants from the consultation, and

I found this to be the trickiest one of the points making up the ICE acronym. It is important for the patient's needs to be met as much as possible, but sometimes their requests are unrealistic or even impossible to achieve within a 10-minute GP consultation. Some are outside the scope of medical practice altogether.

This can be difficult for both the patient and the clinician. It's like trying to reassure a patient that you will do your best to resolve their piercing infection as soon as possible, but you aren't in a position to arrange for them to receive a full refund from the piercing shop, along with a complimentary tattoo.

All clinical placements start with simple observation, or shadowing as we called it, for the first few days. We would literally shadow our supervisors and other team members, walking behind them, going wherever they went and doing whatever they did.

I had a little chair, likely aimed at children, that I would place in the far corner of the consultation room with a notebook and pen, ready to take notes as I watched Daniel or whoever I was shadowing with the patients. The patients were always asked whether they were happy for me to observe the consultation, or whether they would prefer that I left the room. The GP would meet them in the waiting room prior to their appointment to avoid the patient having to feel awkward in front of me if they chose option two. If they did prefer that I left the room, I would swap places with them and sit in the waiting room instead. Fortunately, I was only ever asked to leave the room a couple of times over the course of the placement, meaning that I got to observe a lot.

Many people can now experience the fly-on-the-wall perspective through TV programmes like *24 hours in A&E* and *GPs: Behind Closed Doors*. But nothing is actually the same as being inside the room, feeling the palpable tension and pressure, laughing alongside the patients as they make jokes and nodding enthusiastically when they turn to ask the student's opinion, despite the fact that they are meant to act like the student isn't there at all.

Shadowing the GPs was invaluable and fascinating, more than I had expected it to be. Each GP that I shadowed had their own unique consultation style and ways. Some adopted a parental role, even if the patients were twice their age. This was skilfully and respectfully done, without taking autonomy from the patient or making them feel patronised. Some patients appeared to love this approach and basked in the fact that someone else was guiding and leading them in matters relating to their health. Other GPs took on more of an advisor role, setting out various management options for the patient and helping them to take control in choosing which would be best for them.

I noticed that the GP's consultation style would change depending on the patient sitting before them. GPs who had built up a relationship with their patients over time developed the skill of determining who preferred hard truths and straight facts, and who responded better to sugar coating. The GPs also knew which of their patients would arrive late, which ones would arrive early, who disliked medication and would need persuasion, and who didn't think it was possible to get better at all without a GP prescription of some sort, even if just for paracetamol.

It was all incredibly fascinating. Even though the GP needed to retain so much medical knowledge, they also had to be able to change faces and approach, depending on who their patient needed them to be at that time.

Despite being my first placement, so I had nothing to compare it to, general practice captivated me from the start. Up until that point, I had not been to my own GP much, apart from to get some help with adolescent acne, so the experience was all very new.

Every 10 minutes, as I sat observing the consultations, the GP and I were presented with a new patient, a new person who had their own story. One could be a newborn baby, in the world only a matter of days, and the next could be 100 years old, having done and seen more things than most people around them.

Despite the calm pace of general practice, there are emergency situations that can catch you off guard. A patient may feel unwell and make a GP appointment, not realising that their symptoms actually constitute a medical emergency, and by the time they arrive in the waiting room, an ambulance needs to be called. Medical emergencies even happen to patients on their way to routine appointments.

I remember one particular morning, a patient entered the room holding a small piece of tissue to the side of his head. A trickle of blood escaped where he was applying pressure and ran down his forehead, settling on his eyelid like a maroon eyeshadow. Behind him was a slightly frantic receptionist who was trying to urge him to sit down as she was worried about how he'd fare on the long walk from the waiting room to Daniel's consultation room. But the patient waved her away with a bloodied hand, insisting that he was fine.

'I suppose you're wondering about my head,' he said to Daniel with a smile as he half sat, half fell into the chair. 'I left my house a little bit later than I wanted to, so I had to pick up the pace walking here so as not to miss my appointment. I know how busy you guys are and didn't want to keep you waiting for little old me. In my rush, I missed a step when crossing the road, fell over and headbutted the ground. Just a mild graze, nothing to worry about.'

As he told us this alarming story, the patient threw his blood-soaked tissue into the general waste bin, and fished out another from the packet of Kleenex in his pocket. The bleeding was heavy, a constant stream with no sign of slowing. I didn't actually see the wound, but Daniel, after gloving up, insisted the patient show him what was under the tissue.

Daniel's sharp intake of breath was enough to tell me that it was serious. Daniel immediately advised the patient that he needed to go to hospital right away for cleaning and closing of the wound, and also for a scan of the head due to his daily dose of warfarin.

'But what about my fungal toenail?' the patient asked, dismayed.

'I will book you another appointment, but right now, my concern is that serious head injury of yours!' replied Daniel.

'OK, if you insist, I'll call my daughter and she can drive me to A&E. Don't go wasting the ambulance on me, save it for a real emergency.'

Daniel asked the worried-looking receptionist, who was still hovering in the doorway, to walk the patient back to the waiting area until his daughter could pick him up. To make sure the man's daughter understood the seriousness and urgency of the situation, Daniel even called her at home.

Once the patient had left the practice, Daniel – with freshly gloved hands – removed the blood-soaked tissues and put them into the orange clinical waste bin, its lid hiding its grisly contents.

'So that we don't scare the rest of the patients,' he said, almost reading my mind. Then he added, 'Plus infection control,' as if suddenly remembering that his role was to teach me good clinical practice.

. . .

The shadowing part of my placement didn't last for as long as I had hoped. I'd enjoyed my front-row seat to observe patient consultations. I'd also enjoyed the fact that as I sat in the corner of the room on my child-sized chair, pretending to be invisible, no-one was expecting anything of me, and I had no real responsibilities.

But as my clinical supervisor wisely said, the longer I stayed in the corner, the harder it would be for me to progress and take up more learning opportunities, which was the whole idea of the placement. After spending a bit of time with Daniel, learning the basics of the medical computer software, along with gaining some pointers and useful advice, I was ready to start seeing real-life patients of my own. Daniel would now take the seat in the corner of the room to observe me, although he managed to procure an adult-sized chair.

Comms lectures had taught my fellow students and me the art of history taking, which in its simplest form is finding out what the patient's problem is, but it was down to us to continue to practise the skill. I had assumed that history taking would be simple, allowing the patient to tell the story of their illness or injury, and I wasn't new to talking to people. This was incredibly naïve of me, as life is never straightforward and linear. It's often complicated, and even messy and chaotic at times, and our bodies are no different. So, encouraging patients to talk about their health took work and it was important to get it right in the best interests of the person sitting before me.

History taking requires developing the right balance

between allowing the patient uninterrupted time to talk, explain why they have booked an appointment and what is ailing them, and asking specific questions to help rule out anything serious or life threatening, whilst narrowing down potential diagnoses. Simultaneously, it means trying to work out the most appropriate clinical examinations, and potentially blood tests and scans, arranging and explaining them all, coming up with a plan and typing the patient's notes, all within the allotted 10-minute appointment time. Rushing any part of the process could result in the patient feeling unheard and the clinician missing out on vital, perhaps even life-or-death information. However, taking too long causes the clinician to run late, affecting every single patient for the rest of the clinic.

This is one of the myriad difficulties with general practice.

After my initial apprehension, I felt positive about my upgrade from the shadowing seat to the GP's swivel chair. This was strategically placed by the computer, but facing the screen at an angle, allowing for both note taking and eye contact with the patient. Whilst the patient was talking, the clinician could be typing, nodding, inserting a well-timed 'hmm' and doing anything else to make the consultation go smoothly. Daniel became my own fly on the wall, observing my skills, on hand to answer any questions from the patient that I struggled with.

I was really grateful to all the patients who not only let me watch their consultations with the GP, but also let me practise on them, observed by Daniel. However, some did struggle with the set up, and whilst they consented to having their consultation carried out by a physician associate student, they still directed all of their thoughts and questions over my right shoulder to Daniel.

I didn't mind, though. I didn't yet have all the answers.

A good consultation always begins with a clear introduction. However, after watching Daniel introduce himself smoothly on countless occasions, taking about two seconds to do so, I had underestimated the fact that everyone already knew what a GP was, but no-one was familiar with my role. At least, not back then.

'Hello, I'm Chloe, the physician associate student,' I would say to each patient, a confident smile on my face disguising my own nerves.

'What's that, then?' the first patient of the day interrupted before I could finish my sentence as he sat down in the chair opposite me.

'A physician associate is a medically trained healthcare professional...' I didn't get far with my carefully rehearsed definition before he interrupted again.

'Is that the fancy new name for a GP? A physician thingy?'

I audibly sighed. My introduction wasn't going as smoothly as I had hoped, and I was very aware of the discreet timer Daniel and I had decided to use for each consultation to practise my time management.

Daniel intervened on my behalf. 'I believe that the role was explained to you when you called and booked your appointment, and we asked if you were happy to see a physician associate student being shadowed by the GP. We also gave you a leaflet about the role when you checked in to read in the reception area. I see that you are holding it right now.'

'Ah yes, I was just testing her,' replied the patient with a toothy smile, a chuckle and a wink. I didn't think that he would become one of my favourites.

The confusion regarding my job role wasn't limited to the patients. On Friday lunchtimes, the clinical staff would have a teaching session in the large meeting room of the GP practice. This teaching was led by various consultants from local hospitals, who would provide an hour on different topics related to their specialty. There was plenty of crossover between general practice and hospital medicine, and it was important that we all stayed up to date with clinical guidelines and medical advances, and worked collaboratively in the best interests of the patients.

And a free lunch is always welcome in my book.

Daniel would kindly make sure to introduce me to the guest consultant. 'This is Chloe, our physician associate student,' would be met with an ahhh and a nod of the head. However, this response sometimes translated to the fact that the consultant had no idea what a physician associate was, but believed they should know, and so didn't want to ask. Sometimes the ahh was more confident, and these consultants usually went on to explain that they had either met or worked with a physician associate.

The latter type of consultant was my favourite.

By this stage, I knew more or less everything there was to know about my role, the career itself when I qualified and the progression, but explaining it seemed to be a more difficult task than it needed to be. Doctors and nurses were the easiest reference points for roles within the healthcare profession, so despite my detailed and all-encompassing definition of a physician associate, ultimately, people just wanted to know whether I was more like a nurse or more like a doctor. And the answer was kind of neither, and kind of both.

At the time, there were not many physician associates around, with only four small cohorts graduating before mine. In the Friday lunchtime teachings, I wasn't sure how much information to volunteer about the role, fixated as I was on the pressure of providing the perfect answer in a room full of GPs watching the conversation unfold. I suspected some of them secretly hoped that my explanation would educate them too.

With every consultant or doctor from a local hospital to whom I could explain my role came the potential to sow the concept in their mind, which might lead to them seeking to take on a physician associate student of their own in the future, or even better, hire one for their clinical teams and specialties. Which is why in my head, my ability to give the perfect answer as to what a physician associate was would seal the fate of the rest of my peers throughout the country. Overly dramatic? Maybe, but it was what I considered to be true at the time.

Luckily for me, the fate of my profession didn't actually lie in my explanation of the job role. My only real responsibility was to get through the course in one piece.

CHAPTER 4

COUNTRY MOUSE

Lions, tigers and bears, along with penguins and a baby elephant, are all remnants of an interesting past relating to where I grew up. Wellingborough, a small leafy town in the heart of Northamptonshire, is where I was born and bred. Interestingly, it was also where my parents grew up, though the Wellingborough of their youth was slightly different to that of my younger brothers and me.

In the 70s, Wellingborough boasted a small zoo, home to some quite large animals, who were free to roam the gardens in the middle of the town centre behind what is now a Morrisons supermarket. As times changed and legislation inevitably tightened, the zoo came to be closed permanently. The finality of the decision was accelerated by a man's questionable decision to sneak into the zoo after dark and creep into the leopard's enclosure, resulting in him being mauled by the big cat and losing his entire arm. Now, the only evidence of zoo animals at this particular site is a handful of life-sized wooden sculptures to commemorate its Jumanji-like past.

The primary school that my siblings and I attended was the same one that our dad had been to when he was a little boy, and the secondary school was the same as my mum's. My brothers and I didn't attend these schools in order to continue a grand family tradition, like those who grace the halls of Eton and Harrow, with their names carved onto wooden plaques generation after generation. They were just close by and convenient.

Warwick Primary School was immediately next door to the house where we lived, which provided benefits like not having to wake up as early as my friends to allow time to journey into school. I was also allowed to see myself to school from a young age, giving me an impression of adult maturity as I walked the three-minute journey with my mum watching and waving from the doorstep.

My secondary school, Wrenn, was further away, allowing me the freedom and potential for adventure that early teens desire. Each morning on the walk to school, I observed the ritual of knocking for my friends along the way. Whether they lived on the route or involved a massive detour, it didn't matter. The camaraderie between us was similar to that of Frodo Baggins and his support team in *Lord of the Rings*. No-one got left behind, even if one of us was late, overslept, or couldn't decide which random piece of jewellery was essential for the day of learning.

We were known to the local shopkeepers along the way, who all understood our need for the 10p extra-long strawberry laces to sustain us on our trek to school. Our journey home was equally fun, with the added bonus of spontaneity, particularly in the spring and summer months. It could involve an impromptu water fight, a shopping trip, walking around a park or gathering in a friend's bedroom, all the while avoiding the homework our teachers had set out.

My group of friends stayed more or less the same throughout primary and secondary school. However, for sixth form, I went to a school in a different town, away from the friends that I'd known since infancy. Over time, I started to lose touch with a lot of them as I made new friends. And then the cycle started again as from sixth form, we all went to different universities around the country.

At the time I applied for the postgraduate physician associate course, it was only available at two universities: St George's in London and Aberdeen in Scotland. As I'd grown up in a little town, both London and Aberdeen seemed like magical faraway lands to me.

I decided to apply to both the universities, though by the time I was invited for my interview at Aberdeen, I had already been offered a place at St George's University of London. After discussions and deliberations, I decided to accept my place at St George's University, graciously and gratefully declining that of Aberdeen.

At the time of applying, I had thought that Aberdeen

would be the winner if it came down to choosing between the two universities. However, in the end, the ease with which I could travel home, coupled with the thrill of living in the capital city of England, enticed me more. Wellingborough, though small and insignificant in many respects, still had a direct train line into central London, taking only 50 minutes. At this point in my life, I felt more than ready to spread my wings and fly, but ideally with easy access back home as and when I needed it. I was very much a homebody, after all, a creature of habit with a preference for familiarity.

Whilst I only had two brothers, my wider family was a large one. With more aunts, uncles and cousins than I could count on my fingers and toes, plus grandparents, my family tree was something of a giant sequoia. A couple of aunts lived in Jamaica and Canada respectively, some cousins were in Ireland and some in Luton, but the rest of us lived in the same town. We might have varied in complexion, religion, shape, size, personality and career path, but we were a close family.

It wasn't long before it dawned on me, I would soon be moving away from my hometown, with its 75,000 residents, to London, in which nearly 9 million people were living. I would be leaving friends and family for pastures new, an awfully big step that would involve much upheaval, in order to pursue a career I had only recently found out existed.

So, what are physician associates? They are healthcare professionals who are trained to the medical model and work within a multidisciplinary team under a doctor's supervision. The multidisciplinary team can vary significantly depending on the clinical specialty, but can include doctors of different specialties, surgeons, nurses, healthcare assistants, pharmacists, physiotherapists, and many other amazing members of the wider healthcare profession. At the time of writing, physician associates have been part of the NHS workforce for well two decades, though it is still generally considered a young and new profession.

Before informing my family and friends about my change of career path from something I had planned to do for most of my life to something they would likely never have heard of, I read and learned as much about the profession of physician associate as possible so I would be ready to answer questions and explain all that I could. If I did this well, all who heard me would be cheering me on, fighting an urge to hoist me on to their shoulders and dance me around the room. My family have always been supportive of me, my big ideas and even my flights of fancy. I never doubted their support, but I wanted everyone to be as excited as I was currently feeling.

'Chloe wants to be a doctor' was a line that slipped easily off my parents' tongues whenever they were asked by interested peers. They weren't bragging or boasting, just repeating a story that I had been telling them and myself for years. It was a simple, straightforward and easy-to-understand linear career path.

Then came 'Chloe wants to be a physician associate.' This was less straightforward and harder to understand.

Most people didn't know what a physician associate was, so its declaration lacked clarity.

As a lifelong reader, I know sometimes, the best stories are a bit more complicated. So, I was able to explain the role and the reason behind my change in career, and sell it well. No, I wasn't going to be a doctor, but a physician associate is still a valued member of the healthcare team who examines and treats patients day to day. No, I would not have the title Dr, but I would still study on a medical course and fulfil my lifelong passion to practise medicine and help patients.

Receiving smiles and nods of approval from my friends and family alike, I had passed the test – the first of many to come.

Despite visiting London a few times for day trips and tourist experiences, I wasn't very familiar with it and needed to prepare myself to become a permanent resident. As I was a postgraduate who had already completed undergraduate study, student finance was unavailable to me. Instead, a government career development loan would help me fund my studies. As I had worked at my local hospital for most of the time on my undergraduate degree, I had some savings in the bank, and was fortunate that my parents were able to help financially, too.

I was thankful for all this as I needed all the financial help I could get my hands on. The first year that I would study the postgraduate physician associate course was also the year that tuition fees tripled across the country. With my budgets written out on a piece of paper and my calculator in hand – the same scientific calculator as I'd used in year seven of secondary school, these things never die – I worked out what I would be able to afford to spend on accommodation, rent and bills.

House- and flat-sharing websites and apps provided me with a wealth of knowledge about London rentals, highlighting how naïve I really was. I quickly learned that the rent on a single room in most areas of the capital city would be more expensive than mortgage repayments on a reasonably sized house back in Wellingborough. I learned that the combination of letters and numbers that made up certain London postcodes immediately disqualified the average person from being able to afford to live there, even if they planned never to buy a single thing again.

On the other hand, I learned that some house shares were incredibly affordable, regardless of postcode. But there was always a catch. These arrangements varied in nature, but were generally offered by people who had extra space in their homes and needed a favour in return. Sometimes, it was help with childcare, tutoring, walking pets, house sitting... the list was endless. Although some of these arrangements appeared quite attractive, I refused to burden myself with extra responsibility. If the postgraduate university experience was to be anything like being an undergraduate, it would come with as many academic challenges, and likely plenty more of them. I wanted to give the course my full attention.

There was one property that caught my attention almost straight away. It was a one-bedroom flat in Tooting Broadway with very affordable rent – the price was the same as the flat-sharing places I'd seen. From the pictures included on the online ad, the flat appeared modern and clean with a good-sized bedroom, living room, bathroom and kitchen. It had been listed for a couple of weeks, which wasn't long, but rang some alarm bells. It was such good value for money, why was it still available? Why hadn't it yet been snapped up.

I contacted the landlord who invited me for a viewing. The place was as described and the pictures had given a good representation of it, which I had been cautious about. I failed to see the issue, though deep down, I knew there must be one.

'This is the bedroom, as shown in the pictures,' the landlord said as he continued showing me around. 'Which we will be sharing...' he added more quietly.

'I'm sorry, pardon?' I asked, certain that I had either misheard or suffered from a classic dyslexic misunderstanding.

'As I mentioned in the ad, I will be living here too. We will be flat sharing and room sharing. You will have the double bed and I will sleep on a pull-out bed over there.' He calmly pointed to the space below the alcove window, smiling as if he could read my mind and was trying to reassure me. I didn't know what to say, but I knew one thing: this arrangement wasn't for me. It wasn't how I wanted to live and I wasn't even prepared to entertain the notion.

'Thank you, but I must have misunderstood your ad,' I said. 'I thought you were renting out the entire place.'

'But the ad did mention there'd be a tenant in situ.'

'Yes, but I thought that meant me, that I would be the tenant in situ.' I laughed, realising my mistake, hoping he wouldn't be annoyed. Thankfully, he laughed too.

'Well, if you change your mind, let me know. For some reason, I'm not having as much interest as I thought I would. In fact, you've been the only person to come and view the place.'

Luckily, not too long afterwards, I found a promising place, free from any hidden loopholes or secret room sharers. I saw the advert the first day that it was posted on the SpareRoom website and tracked the necessary Google map route to see how easy or difficult it would be to get to university each day. Happy with the travel arrangements, I then contacted the owner immediately.

The house was large. It had four bedrooms and was home to a lovely family of three: a mother and her two daughters, who were around my own age. The mother had decided to rent out the spare room, and when I compared the price she was asking to similar rooms available in the same area, it was a steal.

I communicated with the landlady Laura, for a little while, asking all the relevant questions whilst simultaneously trying to get a feel for her personality and character. Then as soon as I was able, I travelled to London from Wellingborough to view the place.

I found the house easily. After ringing the doorbell, I

was greeted and ushered inside by a middle-aged woman with a kind face and a ready smile that made her eyes sparkle. This was Laura, and I warmed to her straight away.

It was the same day that Usain Bolt broke the 100 metres world record in the London 2012 Olympic Games. Midway through telling her a little about myself, I was politely interrupted.

'Do you mind if I just watch this race?' Laura asked. 'It's Usain Bolt, it won't take long.'

And, of course, it didn't. Only 9.63 seconds, to be exact.

Once the race was finished and her cheers had subsided, Laura continued. 'So, if you like us, and you like the place, you're welcome to move in any time.' I'd only been in her house five minutes at this point for a whistle-stop tour so quick, it could have given Mr Bolt some competition. After Usain's victory, she did give me a slower more detailed tour, but I had already noted that the atmosphere was warm and inviting, and I knew this woman's home would be somewhere that I could also call home for the time being.

Laura's house was situated just off a busy main road, set on a steep hill. It was quiet, though clearly not free of the parking problems often associated with London living. That didn't affect me as I had decided to sell my little car before moving to the city.

The house was close enough to St George's for a morning stroll into university each day, though far enough that if I accidentally forgot something, I wouldn't want to go back to fetch it, so at home it would stay. Unless it was my phone. I would have swum across the Thames to retrieve my phone. St George's University is in Tooting Broadway, Southwest London, near the end of the Northern Line. This was far off the beaten track in comparison to all of my previous London trips.

The journey to London when I moved into my new accommodation was a tight squeeze in my dad's car. Dad drove, my nan decided to come along for the ride, and I was squashed in too, along with everything that I felt was essential, which was the entire contents of my bedroom. But I was incredibly excited. This was my first time moving away from home and not just to anywhere, but to London. I was also nervous and apprehensive. Leaving the comfort of home is scary for everyone, but I was still learning and finding out about myself in light of the new diagnosis of SpLDs.

After a long and tedious journey, we arrived at Tooting Broadway. In Wellingborough, the weather had been warm and pleasant, but London felt like the Tropics in comparison. I soon came to realise that London is always slightly warmer than Wellingborough. It's only by a couple of degrees, but it would feel like the climate of a different country each time I went back home to visit.

As soon as the traffic allowed us, we crossed slowly over to the SW17 postcode. I was in awe. The colours, the vibrancy, the cultures were demonstrated not only by the people, but also the shops, restaurants and languages. Young people, older people, walking along the streets of Tooting Broadway, chatting enthusiastically and cheerfully in many different tongues.

The vast amount of people on the streets was something that I wasn't used to, except when Wellingborough was holding its annual street carnival and procession. Today, it was Saturday lunchtime in the peak of summer, but still, in comparison to the town I had just left behind, the hustle and bustle was remarkable. At first, I was convinced that there must be something going on. Maybe the shops had been forced to evacuate or were practising a fire drill, causing all these people to pile on to the streets. But I soon realised that this was just a typical Saturday in Tooting Broadway.

I had never before been to a place that catered to Caribbean, African, Asian, and European tastes and cuisines. Sourcing haircare products for my naturally thick afro would no longer be a struggle nor a chore; the options were minimal back home. In Tooting Broadway, the local beauty shop supplied brands that I had only seen whilst visiting family in America or Canada. Now, moments from where I was living, I had access to more premium hair and beauty products than I could carry (or afford).

I had never before felt so included, despite being an absolute stranger.

. . .

It wasn't uncommon to hear rumours that London was so expensive, you could barely afford to live. Whilst I had verified this in regards to property, wondering how people could afford a home of their own, to my relief, it didn't affect my modest student expenditure in other ways. The prices of food and other essentials were the same as back home.

Tooting Broadway was home to a large indoor market. Whilst I loved to frequent it, each time I visited, I feared that I would never be able to find the way out. To me, it bore a close resemblance to a rabbit warren, with the added bonus of entrances and exits appearing to change position at random. I never exited the same way that I entered, but each time, I was just grateful to find any way out.

Unlike Wellingborough, which gifted my senses during the summer months with the aromas of freshly cut grass and flowers in full bloom along the roadside, in parks and in gardens, London offered the warm and slightly overpowering fug of car fumes and pollution, greeting me aggressively as I stepped on to the main road. The pavements were noticeably darker, not due to different coloured concrete slabs, but because of dirt. Everyone seemed to smoke, a habit that was noticeably going out of style in Wellingborough, and there must have been a crisis every five seconds. The screeching sound of sirens was never ending, although living in close proximity to a hospital would account for the high number of ambulances. It didn't, however, explain the equally high number of police cars and fire engines that would whizz up and down the high street throughout the day.

Back in Wellingborough, if an ambulance or police car sped past, I'd stop to consider the situation, wondering what emergency was unfolding ahead and hoping that the people involved would be OK. Then, after a brief moment of reflection, I would carry on with my day. In London, if I stopped every time I heard a siren, I would never move. It wasn't long before I had heard so many sirens, I stopped hearing them altogether.

One thing that I didn't foresee in light of my diagnosis was having so much difficulty navigating in and around London. I should have considered this, but growing up in a small town meant I'd never needed to learn how to read a map. As a child, I was taken to different places by my parents, unaware that I was unconsciously becoming familiar with pretty much the entire town. I knew where the roads led, so when I learned to drive, I could navigate my way around independently.

Living in Southwest London, away from my family and hometown, I had a keen interest to explore my new city. However, it soon made me realise how much I had taken for granted the fact that I knew how to get around without a second thought in Wellingborough. I quickly learned the route to and from the university, but it was very straightforward – luckily, as any journey that deviated from my ideal straight line often resulted in frustration. Whether I was on foot, the bus, or the Tube, it didn't matter. There was no method of travel that provided better results. Even though I knew full well by this point that I was dyslexic and dyscalculic, it still had a funny way of creeping up and surprising me with newfound confusion, difficulties and frustrations.

Like anyone in a new area, I relied heavily on navigation apps, but for me, these didn't provide the clarity I needed. For someone with dyslexia, the navigation instructions require further interpretation. Despite my best efforts, I could never work out the direction that I needed to be travelling to arrive at my desired destination. Sometimes, the blue arrow on the app would show me that I was walking in the right direction, then halfway along the road, I would realise that I was actually walking away from where I wanted to be going. A stranger directing me to go left or right was pointless, particularly at a crossroads where I had only a 50/50 chance of getting it correct.

The bus stops in Wellingborough are nicely spaced out and named after the street they are on. This couldn't work in London due to the bus stops being so close to each other, many situated on the same street. Instead, each bus stop is given letters to identify it. This might seem straightforward enough, but the lettering doesn't always make sense or go in any sort of logical order. At least, not to me. If I needed to board a specific bus at stop x, I'd often realise it was actually round the corner on a road that I hadn't even noticed.

Another issue was not knowing the direction I needed to be travelling in, and consequently not knowing which side of the street to be on to catch the right bus. Unlike back home, where the roads were often quiet and deserted, I found it almost impossible to cross the busy London roads. The need to look out simultaneously for cars, buses, bikes, scooters, even skateboarders passing in both directions, whilst trying to see if my bus was approaching, or worse waiting to leave without me, was more than I had bargained for. I found myself relying on my new friend, the pedestrian crossing green man, to get me safely across. Helpfully, inside the buses in London, the name of the next stop was clearly displayed, so if I realised I was on the right bus but going in the wrong direction, I could easily press the bell, get off, cross the road and try again.

When it came to the Tube, one of my saving graces was that Tooting Broadway is so near to the end of the Northern Line, I would most likely be travelling northbound. It is also as nice and simple as an underground station can be as there are only two platforms. At the bottom of the escalator, I could either turn left for the southbound train and the end of the line, or turn right for the northbound line into central London towards popular landmarks, museums, galleries and, most frequented by me, London St Pancras station to catch the train home to see my family.

It is true, though, that I still got on the wrong platform and headed in the wrong direction more than once. Even though I took screenshots and even handwrote my journey step by step, it just never seemed to go as planned, and lack of internet access whilst underground did me no favours. I was heavily reliant on the little free paper underground maps that used to be provided at each station and would have at least five crumpled at the bottom of my bag at any given time.

Over time, travel did get easier. Due to the magic of repetition, I grew more confident and less remorseful at my errors. In London, everyone is so busy and focused on their own thing, so it didn't matter if I went the wrong way. No-one really knew apart from me. It wasn't long before I was strutting through the stations like I owned them rather than cowering in fear, as if a wrong turn meant I would be trapped underground forever.

Small wins to most people, but big wins for me.

CHAPTER 5

SPEED DATING

I haven't personally participated in speed dating but understand the general premise of it. You have a short amount of time to hold a conversation with someone you have only just met. When the allotted time is up, you move on to the next person and start the conversation all over again. At the end of the event, you identify any dates that went particularly well and the people who you wish to meet again.

Clinical placements reminded me of this. They were a test of compatibility. I put my best face forward, spent some time checking to see if there was any chemistry between me and the specialty. Sometimes, I knew straight away that it was not going to lead to anything serious, but I saw it through to the end.

Some of my colleagues started their clinical placement rotations already knowing which specialty they were looking forward to the most, or even where they were planning on working after qualifying. Others, like myself, were just keeping an open mind and giving every specialty a fair chance, seeing if a love connection happened.

When it comes to my environment, whether working or personal, routine and familiarity help me to navigate and minimise the confusion, stress and discomfort that having a dyslexic brain can bring. The revolving door of clinical placements, however, was anything but routine and familiar. The ever-changing nature of the journeys to each hospital, clinical specialties, colleagues and teams throughout my physician associate course was something that I found difficult, before I'd even added in the drama of all the knowledge that I needed to learn. As soon as I started to feel settled and comfortable within the specialty, it would be time to say goodbye, move on to the next placement and learn the ropes all over again.

Despite preferring the comfort of familiarity, I knew that the changes were good for me. When else would I be able to experience working as a physician associate in numerous clinical specialties? Each one taught me more and more about medicine, but also a surprising amount about myself.

There were many times that I wished my brain functioned just like everyone else's around me and that I was normal. But what is normal? There is so much beauty and identity to be found in being unique. I didn't just go along with the crowd or maintain the status quo as typically, my preferences and the way I worked differed to other people's, encouraging me to constantly form my own path and do what worked best for me, even if it meant doing it alone.

Whilst academia continued to be a constant struggle for me, my ability to communicate, connect and empathise with patients came naturally. Patients warmed to me, and I to them, even if I wasn't able to regurgitate my medical textbook word for word, like some of my classmates.

A&E was a placement I wasn't sure whether I was excited or nervous for. Mine took place at Yellow Hospital, modern and busy hospital that was easy to get to on the train from where I lived – once I worked out the nearest station, as it was very close to two stations, with one being much more straight forward to get to the hospitals front doors.

Before starting each placement, we physician associate students would spend some time in class, preparing the basics of what we needed to know in advance. TV programmes like *Casualty* and *Holby City*, which I had enjoyed from a young age, were now my only points of reference for the A&E department. This didn't really help me much at all. I was unaware, for example, that the department was split into three wards: minors, majors and resuscitation (or resus, as we called it).

After a patient is triaged upon entering the A&E department, which means gathering necessary information to determine how much of an emergency their medical problem really is, that's when it's decided whether they should be treated in minors, majors or resus. Occasionally, paramedics call the A&E department from the ambulance en route to the hospital to inform the staff there if the patient they have just collected will need to go straight into resus or majors. This means the medical staff can ensure everything is ready and be on hand as soon as the ambulance arrives with the critically ill patient.

My A&E placement was shared with a few of my classmates. Despite having enjoyed spending my GP placement alone, I soon found out that there were many benefits to being with my fellow physician associate students. On one occasion, I was asked if I wanted to slot a dislocated shoulder back into its socket – under the guidance of the supervising consultant, of course. At the time, I couldn't think of anything worse, so looked pleadingly in the direction of a classmate. Picking up on my cue, he enthusiastically volunteered to give it a go, whilst I discreetly slunk off to another part of the ward, almost certain that I wouldn't even be able to stomach observing.

A rota ensured my colleagues and I were getting an equal amount of time on the three areas of A&E, all with valuable and unique learning experiences on offer. The rota also meant that my classmates and I had plenty of individual learning opportunities, although we made sure to meet up for lunch in the hospital canteen and swap stories of the morning's horrors and fascinations.

Alongside the physician associate students doing their placement in the department, there were also nursing and medical students. I always found it interesting working with other clinical students, if sometimes a little daunting. Physician associate was a new profession, so patients and staff often didn't really know where we fitted into the multidisciplinary team of the NHS workforce. I had heard rumours of some medical students being hostile to physician associate students whilst sharing a placement, perhaps because they believed we would be stepping on their toes or taking learning and working opportunities away from them. I personally didn't experience any hostility towards the profession during my time as a student and was keen to demonstrate to those who were unsure how useful a physician associate could be to a clinical team. We all shared the same end goal, after all: providing good patient care.

One of the most interesting things I learned about myself on my minors A&E placement was that I wasn't as hardy, resilient and immune from being adversely affected by anything unsavoury I witnessed as I had previously believed. It wasn't pouring blood, oozing, infected wounds, projectile vomit or any other bodily fluids or solids that made me feel woozy. It was actually something far less dramatic: broken bones.

Whilst I was on my A&E placement, a patient came into the department with a netball injury which had occurred only an hour or so beforehand. Somewhere between the patient attempting to obstruct the ball, colliding with her opponent, and falling awkwardly onto the concrete ground, she'd injured her wrist. In addition to being bruised and swollen, it was clearly sitting at an awkward angle.

The patient had consented to being seen by a student, so I took her history and started to gently examine her wrist. I was feeling slightly uneasy, though unsure why. I pinpointed where the patient's pain was, and then discussed her medical case with my clinical supervisor, who agreed with my plan to arrange an X-ray.

The X-ray report came back much more quickly than I had expected, even though it was a quiet midweek morning, so I shouldn't have been too surprised. On the side wall of the A&E department was a box, a little bigger than an A4 piece of paper, its purpose to illuminate the X-ray pictures, making them easier to interpret. My clinical supervisor held up my netball patient's X-ray against the illuminated box and asked me for my thoughts.

I was still trying to understand and master X-ray interpretation in my personal study time. With slightly squinted eyes and tilted head, I observed the patient's wrist bones on the X-ray. They somewhat resembled a dinner fork, something I had recently read to look out for, which pointed to a diagnosis of Colles fracture. This is a common injury resulting from falling on to outstretched hands.

I told my supervising consultant that I thought it was a Colles fracture. Instead of being a little smug for answering correctly so quickly, though, I felt an intense heat rising through my body, heard a whooshing in my ears, and saw black spots appear before my eyes.

I was going to faint.

I refused to succumb to my horizontal fate, so plonked myself down on to a nearby chair, putting my head between my knees, willing myself to get over this, and quickly. My patient was waiting for me behind a cubicle curtain.

My consultant supervisor, visibly concerned, asked me if I was OK as he handed me a plastic cup of water. I reassured him that I was fine and likely just dehydrated, which wasn't completely untrue. I never drank enough. But I knew that the more I looked at either the X-ray of the broken bones or the patient's awkwardly hanging wrist, the less likely it was that I would remain upright and conscious.

After taking a few moments, sipping the tepid water and declining the offer either to be checked over inside one of the free A&E cubicles or to go home early, I decided to hand over my patient to one of the nurses. She would take my patient off to get her wrist put into a plaster cast that she would wear for the next six weeks. That was something I had really wanted to see as I had always wondered how the casts were put on, particularly the brightly coloured ones that people occasionally turned up wearing following some accident at school, but I didn't yet trust my faculties and thought it was better that I didn't push it.

I did wonder whether this reaction would turn out to be an isolated one-off incident. However, over the course of my A&E placement, anytime I saw a fractured, broken or displaced bone, even on X-ray, my pulse would start to rise and my face would feel clammy. If I ignored the signals that my body was giving me, it wouldn't end well.

I wasn't alone in this weirdly specific aversion, though. One of the nurses working in the department couldn't take the smell of blood. Not the sight of it, just the rich, irony smell. If there was so much blood on or coming out of a patient that the smell became overwhelming, she too would find herself sitting on a chair, bent over with her head between her legs.

There were other members of staff who just couldn't handle bodily fluids of any kind. Dealing with them wouldn't necessarily make them faint, but they did have an extremely strong aversion to vomit, urine etc. Working previously as a healthcare assistant on a male stroke ward had more than equipped me to deal with these particular delights and given me a noteworthy resilience, provided I had on tight-fitting gloves, a long apron and shoes that I didn't care too much about.

Although quiet at times (for only a matter of minutes), the A&E minors department was never boring. Some patients attended in wild fancy dress costumes after sustaining an injury at a cosplay event. Some attended not dressed at all. Sometimes people were keen to share their story of bravery and bravado, whereas others by their very demeanour told me they wanted to be asked no questions about what had led them to the department.

One patient, despite agreeing to be seen by a student, was particularly shy and embarrassed, having sustained her injury under circumstances that you might not expect from an 83-year-old woman. I eventually persuaded her to reveal that she had been attempting a seductive bedroom routine for her husband, which involved part dance and part role play, all in stiletto heels. Unfortunately, she had lost her balance and taken a small tumble, luckily on to the bed, resulting in no more than a sprain. Her husband, who had accompanied her to hospital, told me he thought she'd better get checked out 'due to her age'. From her glare, I could see that she didn't appreciate the sentiment. Nor did she appreciate being rushed out of the house without first being allowed to change into more appropriate daywear.

There were people who really didn't need to attend A&E at all. One came in with a small splinter in the tip of her finger. I took her history, examined the area, and then confidently removed the splinter from her finger with my gloved hand, handing it back to her as a souvenir. After ensuring there was nothing else on her mind that she wished to discuss, I kindly and gently explained to the patient that her A&E visit was neither an accident nor an emergency, and therefore not a proper use of the service. She could have removed the little splinter by herself with minimal effort. Though at the same time, the feeling of being solely in charge of this patient, completely fixing her problem and clearing her with my supervisor for discharge, was great. I felt like a superhero, even if it was just for removing a splinter.

After stitching, casting, bandaging, treating and advising people in minors, we were generally able to send them back home again to continue with their lives as if A&E was just a pit stop in their day. Majors and resus, however, wouldn't be anywhere near as straightforward.

On my first day of shadowing in resuscitations, we had no patients on the small ward with only two or three beds. This was very different to minors, which resembled a conveyor belt of people entering and being discharged constantly throughout the day. I was disappointed that there were no patients, but my supervisor reassured me that the calm wouldn't last.

Whilst it was quiet, we used the time to talk about the department and how it worked. Then she showed me the different equipment and emergency medications in case I needed to help in the event of an emergency. She and the resuscitations team were not expecting me to perform any life-saving procedures, but if they had to ask me to call for help, bleep a clinician, or even gather equipment, I would need to know how to do it and what to gather. I was grateful for her calm, but the more she talked me through the ward and the type of patients that came in, the more I wondered what I had got myself into. I soon started to wish I was back on minors.

Then it was all go as the first patient of the day was wheeled speedily through the swinging doors and onto the resuscitations ward. A man in his mid-30s, he had fallen from a high ladder and hadn't yet regained consciousness. He was still wearing his work uniform, with the logo on his top telling me that he was a roofer.

He had a few scratches and scrapes on his arms and across his face, on which it appeared he'd landed, but he didn't look as injured as I would have expected. Under different circumstances, he would have looked like he was having a comfortable mid-morning nap.

Being unconscious, he was unable to tell me what hurt, what felt numb, how many fingers I was holding up – valuable questions I'd relied on in minors to take a history. Instead, my supervisor had told me, what was helpful in situations like this was imaging from various scans to identify any broken bones, damaged organs or internal bleeding.

The patient's wife had come in with him, and she was hovering by his bedside, looking frantic. She appeared to be a similar age to him, a decade or so older than myself. Clutching her mobile phone in her hand until her knuckles whitened and still wearing fluffy slippers on her feet, she was firing lots of questions at the doctors and nurses, who were preoccupied with cutting and removing items of clothing and attaching the patient to different machinery and bags of fluids.

Getting no response, the patient's wife came over to me as I stood, wide eyed and feeling small, in the corner of the room, trying to keep out of everyone's way. 'Is he going to be OK?' she asked me desperately in a voice no more than a whisper. I told her that I didn't know, but the team would do their best for him. Then I asked if she wanted some water, which she did, and if she would like to come with me to get it. She nodded.

The water machine was only just outside the door, but we walked out together, side by side in absolute silence. When I'd poured her water and was passing it to her gently, I realised that her free hand was shaking. I wanted to be doing more for her, giving her the information that I could see from her eyes she so desperately needed, and felt a little pathetic only being able to offer her a drink.

As if reading my thoughts, she said, 'Thank you for everything.' I felt like a fraud. I hadn't done anything; the people actually helping her were back on the ward, working on her husband.

'You're welcome,' I said with a warm smile, accepting that what she needed in the moment vs how big I felt my contribution was were likely two very different things.

The patient eventually woke up, and in a very pleasant mood too. I didn't know if his personality was normally playful and jokey, or whether it was the strong pain relief pumping through his veins, but either way, it was lovely to witness his wife's relief. He was later wheeled to another ward on his hospital bed, where his multiple broken bones would be looked after by the orthopaedic team.

On the whole, A&E was a strange place to get used to. One moment it could be really quiet, providing a rare opportunity to speak to the rest of the team and ask how their weekend had been. The next moment, there would be a large influx of patients who needed tending to, some vomiting, some crying, some in pain, some semi-conscious, as if they had all just shared a large coach on a day trip to the hospital. From watching the other clinical staff, I learned that the trick to avoid getting overwhelmed by the sights, sounds and sometimes smells, along with the list of names on the whiteboard of patients waiting to be seen, was just to focus on one at a time.

The acute medical unit (AMU), another placement destination of mine, was similar in its unpredictability. It was an interesting ward as it didn't have a specialty as such. It was made up of patients who had gone through A&E, but needed to spend more time in hospital to get better after their triage and treatment. In that case, they would be transferred on to the AMU ward, until a hospital bed on the ward specifically related to the specialty that covered their ailment, for example cardiology or respiratory, became available. This meant that the patients on AMU varied significantly in age, medical conditions and state of health.

My AMU placement was at Pink Hospital. The ward

was deceptively large from the outside as all I could see through the windows was a long, wide corridor. It was only once I walked along the corridor that I saw it opened to the left and right on to multiple bays and side rooms. It had a typical ward smell: a not terrible combination of cleaning chemicals and air freshener.

Some of the patients on the AMU were transferred to their specialty ward quite quickly, only just getting comfortable before they were wheeled off again. On other occasions, a patient would stay on the AMU ward for weeks, even months. This could be for many reasons, one of the more frequent being that the patient actually improved in health, so wasn't unwell enough to be sent to the specialty ward, but wasn't well enough to be discharged back home without help. Carers or home adjustments like rails, bathroom modifications and stair-lifts were sometimes required and could take a while to arrange. Whilst this was being organised, the patient stayed in hospital. It was the safer option, but I couldn't help wondering if it was the best use of resources.

For the patients waiting to be transferred to their specialty ward, the specialist teams who would be looking after them would come down to AMU to review them. This meant that although AMU had its own team of doctors, nurses and healthcare staff, there were frequently also other teams from around the hospital on the ward.

Each morning, AMU had a ward round, like all departments. This was where a group of clinicians, typi-cally a consultant, registrar, other doctors, nurses and students, would move from bed to bed to review each patient and make a plan for their treatment that day. Sometimes, medications would need to be added, stopped or tweaked, blood tests arranged, or other forms of clinical management provided.

I hadn't actually been a part of ward rounds before starting the physician associate course. When I worked as a healthcare assistant, I only covered the late afternoon shift, so missed them taking place. We had mock ward rounds at the university, so by the time our placements began, we understood the gist of them, but this was my first experience of the real thing.

Even though I was sure I'd merely be a spectator of the group, ward rounds did make me a little nervous. I had heard stories of keen consultants who wanted to give students in their departments opportunities to both learn and demonstrate their knowledge, and they did this by firing questions at them. Although the consultants were rooting for the students and encouraging them to get the answers right, this was a nightmare of mine all the same, particularly in front of the patient that I would be helping to look after all day. They might see the crack in my façade and realise I didn't know what I was doing after all.

One particular morning, I arrived slightly late for the AMU ward round due to the train being delayed. I saw a team of clinical staff going from bed to bed and was relieved that I could slip to the back of the group with my lateness going unnoticed.

I followed the ward round for a while, but became a

little confused when the group all left the ward together and started off down the main hospital corridor, deep in conversation. I didn't want to interrupt or ask any questions, but when we arrived at a completely different ward, I decided to speak up.

'Erm, is this the AMU ward round?' I asked. The others all turned to look at me in surprise, likely unaware that I had even been following behind them, then one by one, they started to laugh. They found it extremely humorous, but were all very kind and explained that I had tagged on to the wrong ward round. The AMU team were... well, back in the AMU.

With my pink stethoscope bobbing around my neck, I hurried back to my ward. I found my supervising consultant and explained what had happened. He found it equally entertaining, as did the rest of the team who he insisted on sharing the story with.

I made sure going forward to always check which team I was with when doing the ward rounds.

At the time of my clinical placement, the AMU ward had Caleb, its very own fully fledged and qualified physician associate, on the team. This was unusual back then as the role was still so new. What it meant for me was that a lot of my learning and clinical experiences came from an actual physician associate showing me first-hand how the role fits into the ward and the types of things that he would do within the department day to day. It also meant that I didn't have to spend so much time each day explaining to patients and staff exactly what a physician associate was, as Caleb had already done the groundwork for me.

'Hello, I'm Chloe, the physician associate student working on the ward for the next few weeks,' would usually get the enthusiastic response, 'Ah yes, a Caleb! Welcome to AMU.'

The AMU was one of my longer placements, lasting 12 weeks, with the rest only being three weeks. This gave me a chance not only to really get to know the AMU team, who were varied, fun and humorous characters, but also to develop my hands-on clinical skills, like taking venous blood samples.

On one particular morning, there was a ward announcement that our usual phlebotomist was unavailable, and we would need to take our own blood samples from patients. One of the ward registrars, Zec, had decided to take me under his wing. He came over to find me and asked excitedly if I wanted to take the blood samples from all the patients that morning for a chance to practise.

'I would love to, but I haven't yet had any success.' I replied. 'I've done the reading, practiced at University but have never been successful at collecting a blood sample from a real human.'

'No way!' he replied in an animated fashion, as if I was telling a joke and he was choosing to play along. When he realised that I wasn't in fact joking, he made it his mission for the rest of the day to help me practise taking blood until I had mastered it.

Zec was originally from South Sudan and had a darkish skin complexion, similar to my own. In a lot of the reading I had done around taking blood samples, the textbooks and online articles advised me to look out for the large, chunky blue-green veins in the patient's elbow crease. What I hadn't considered was that with darker skin, I wouldn't be able to see this vein as it's not visible as described. Zec taught me that the best way to take a blood sample, contrary to what I had previously read, was to use gloved fingers to feel for the vein, not just rely on looking for it with my eyes.

After Zec had fetched a small clinical trolley filled with an array of equipment that he thought we might need, such as different sized needles, butterfly needles, cotton wool, tape and little round plasters, perfect for covering needle punctures, we sat at the doctor's station, me with maximum concentration and my notebook at the ready.

'You won't be needing that,' he said. 'Taking notes won't help you, only practising will.' With a comical flourish, he took my notebook and pen from my hands and placed them down next to the bench where I was sitting. Then he laid his arm on the desk and, after showing me how to put on the tourniquet and tighten it, helped me locate the best veins. I told him that historically, my veins had been difficult to find when I'd had blood samples taken. He seemed excited about this and taught me how and where to find my own best chunky veins for easy blood taking.

'OK, ready to give it a go? I want you to try and get flashbacks of blood into this butterfly needle,' he said with a smile on his face, presenting his arm to me like a gift. 'Flashback' was a term which meant, when a specific needle was in the vein, you would see a little bit of blood at the top of the needle tube. When the blood travelled into the tube, it confirmed that you were in the right place.

After plenty of practice and many failed attempts, the registrar's arm was covered with so many spot plasters, he looked like he had lost a fight with a porcupine, but I'd got the hang of it. The ward was quiet, so every now and again a member of the team would come over to us and ask what we were doing. Zec explained that he was helping me to master the art of venous blood-sample taking and we were open to more volunteer arms, which immediately made them scuttle away again.

To be honest, I didn't blame them. Regardless of how passionate a clinical educator or supervisor I was to become in the future, I'm not sure that I would have been brave enough to present my arm to a first timer for blood taking, like a lamb to the slaughter.

Unfortunately, some patients never left the AMU ward in this life, and it was here that I experienced my first patient death. It happened towards the end of my 12-week placement, by which time I had grown tremendously in both confidence and skill.

An elderly gentleman had been admitted on to the ward alone. We were still gathering his medical notes together to learn more about him, but in the meantime, he needed to have a catheter fitted to help him pass urine as he wasn't well enough to get out of bed. I volunteered.

I proudly wheeled my trolley of equipment to his bed space, drawing the curtains around us, confident that as I had done it a few times before, I would be able to catheterise this patient easily and uneventfully. I introduced myself to him and explained what I wanted to do, checking that he was happy for me to proceed. The patient seemed to be hovering between wakefulness and sleep, but with his eyes closed, he whispered his consent.

I tried to engage him in conversation as I started the task, but he remained quiet. He looked comfortable enough, though. After opening everything that I needed and placing it on the trolley, I told him that I was going to uncover him slightly, and as I did so, the patient let out a big sigh. The sigh wasn't an unusual response, particularly if the patient was shy; what was unusual was the way his hand fell heavily from the bed rail where it had been resting and his body stiffened slightly and rolled off the right-hand side. His chest was no longer rising and falling through his hospital gown and I could feel no breath escaping as I held my trembling hand over his mouth.

I'd had recent basic and advanced life-support training, but still froze on the spot, wide eyed and confused.

Part of me wanted to push the red emergency button on the wall, as we were advised to do at times like this. The other part of me was worried about people seeing the patient exposed, as I respected his dignity. It would have been easy just to cover the patient and press the emergency button, but I was unable to think straight. Instead, I called for Caleb, the qualified physician associate on the ward, like my life depended on it. I'm sure my cry terrified the patients on the other side of the curtain.

Caleb had informed me he would be close by if I needed him during the catheterisation, and true to his word, he rushed in almost instantly. He took one look at the patient and hit the emergency alarm on the wall with a clenched fist. I heard footsteps running towards us from all directions beyond the patient's closed curtain. One person came in with the emergency equipment; one came holding a file containing the patient's notes, which she quickly flicked through. Another pressed the CPR button on the patient's bed, laying it completely flat and closer to the floor. Someone started to attach defibrillation stickers to the patient's chest, but at that point the person holding the patient's notes shouted for us all to stop. She had found a DNAR form at the front of his notes, meaning that he did not want to be resuscitated if his heart stopped.

The doctors and nurses in the patient's bed space thanked each other and dispersed one by one, leaving Caleb and me along with one other doctor and the now-deceased patient. I later learned that thanking everyone for their efforts in a resuscitation attempt, regardless of the outcome, was customary and helped provide a drop of comfort in the difficult situation.

Caleb asked me if I was OK as I stood at the head of the bed, looking down at the patient. Without thinking, I slowly walked out from behind the closed curtains, out of the ward and into the staffroom. I was expecting it to be empty, so as I pushed open the door, I immediately burst into tears before it had even closed behind me. The staffroom, however, was full of people. A patient's relative had just dropped off a big box of chocolates and the staff were ensuring that they got their hands on the best ones first.

Everyone rushed over to me, asking what had happened and telling me to sit down. As Caleb came in behind me, I told them in between sobs that I had killed a patient whilst trying to catheterise him. Caleb quickly jumped in and said that the patient had been very unwell and would have passed away at that moment, whether or not I was attempting to catheterise him. Then someone pushed a fistful of chocolates from the open box into my hand for edible comfort, and this time, I accepted the offer to go home early.

On my way out, one of the junior doctors suggested we did a quick debrief before I left. I would have preferred to do it another day, but almost as if reading my mind, she said that it was better to talk through an incident straight after it had happened to reduce the burden that I would take home at the end of the day. We went to the quiet room and I explained how guilty and horrible I felt. It was as if I had robbed the patient of his dignity in his last moments. If I had known what was about to happen, I would have sat with him, held his hand, told him a peaceful story, even whispered a little prayer, or just been a quiet companion as he breathed his last.

'But Chloe, at least he wasn't alone,' she said.

And I'm glad that he wasn't.

CHAPTER 6

HANDS ON

Before I started to study to become a physician associate, I already knew the random and strange fact that a human head weighs about 10 pounds. I can't recall how I learned this, but it has always stayed with me. As I held the severed head, it felt much lighter than 10 pounds, though it was true that I had no idea what 10 pounds would feel like in my hands.

Another reason why the weight might have felt wrong was that I was actually holding two halves of the head, one in each hand. It had been neatly and carefully cut in two, the head sliced with obvious precision between the eyes, straight through the middle of the nose, and down the perfect centre of its slightly parted lips. There was no skin on the face and no hair on the head. Only the short, dark wisps of eyelashes curled from between the skinless closed eyelids.

The room I was in was large, sparse and cold. It was also underground. All of these features seemed fitting for a dissection room, although the name was a slight misnomer. We did not dissect anything or anyone ourselves. The body parts that were provided for us to examine had already been dissected by students on other courses, such as human anatomy.

There was a pretty short supply of generous individuals who donated their precious bodies after death to help students further their medical learning and careers. This meant that their families had not been able to bury or cremate them with the closure of a funeral service, and would have had to find different ways to commemorate their departure. For this reason above all others, the cadavers, which is what we called the bodies, had to be looked after, respected and distributed fairly between different kinds of clinical students, to ensure that the most benefit could be gained from the individual's selfless act.

I personally didn't mind that I wouldn't get to dissect cadavers first hand. It was hard enough constantly trying not to disappoint the living, let alone adding the pressure of not disappointing the dead with my sweat covered brow and unsteady hand.

I hadn't known what to expect before my first dissection room session. The room itself was a bit of a hidden entity. We accessed it by a secluded staircase, hidden behind heavy double doors. Along the dimly lit corridor at the bottom, we came to the lockers, where we were told to leave all of our belongings as the only things permitted inside of the dissection room were our paper for notes and the questions we needed to answer for our syllabus learning, the thick blue lab coat we were to wear over our clothes, and a pen. For most people, pens had a habit of wandering, and in the dissection room, they would often turn up next to or even resting on various body parts. I was grateful not to be someone who had an instinctive habit of putting the pen in their mouth whilst lost in deep thought.

Once we had put our things into the lockers and hung our coats on the hooks, we were led through a second set of double doors by the session facilitator, and then another set before stepping into the dissection room. The first thing that I noticed was not how bright the room was, particularly in contrast to the dimly lit corridors, but the smell. My brain and vivid imagination had unconsciously made me brace myself for the smell of decomposing bodies, but that wasn't the case. Instead, my nose was assaulted by the potent chemical smell of formaldehyde.

The smell of formaldehyde is hard to describe. It's neither a particularly bad smell nor a particularly pleasant one, but it is powerful and seems to get into your very pores. I often believed I could smell the formaldehyde on my skin for the rest of the day after spending time in the dissection room. It was likely just in my mind, though, as no-one else mentioned any lingering smells.

Head in hands – not my own head, but the two halves

of the cadaver's – I looked around the room at the rest of my classmates. We had formed small groups positioned around shiny silver tables, heads and half heads on each. Each week, the body parts laid out for us would change, like a surprise buffet, to be reflective of whichever systems we had been covering in lectures. Some weeks, the tables would present hearts, some with disease or enlargement, or fatty plaques that the facilitators of the session would be keen to point out. Other times, the tables held lungs, kidneys, hands, feet, chests, torsos, legs and even genitalia. However, each specimen had the same feel to it – cold, firm and stiff – and the same look – white with a faint pinkish tinge from all of the blood having been drained and the skin removed.

To me, St George's University of London was almost the complete opposite of the university I had not long left. The University of Northampton, particularly my campus, was large, open, green and very modern. St George's University of London was smaller, less green and considerably older, but with that came a rich history, including notable alumni dating all the way back to the 18th Century. History was a subject that I had loved in secondary school, and at St George's, I enjoyed looking at the plaques, posters and busts around the site and the hospital, detailing key people and events linked to the university.

Edward Jenner, often referred to as the father of

immunology (Riedel, 2005), was one of the most notable alumni. Originally from rural Gloucestershire, Jenner enrolled at St George's University in 1770, and was a student of another famous alumnus, John Hunter. I wondered whether Jenner would have found the adjustment from small-town life to the crowds of the capital city as much of a shock to the system as I did. At least he wouldn't have had the difficulty of navigating the London Underground system.

After completing his medical training, Jenner went back to Gloucestershire to work as a GP and surgeon. His care covered a huge area of approximately 400 square miles, and was extended even to those without the funds to pay for it.

Around this time, smallpox was a global pandemic, killing millions every year. Even those fortunate enough to survive the disease would often be left blind or scarred. However, Jenner noticed that the local milkmaids didn't seem to be contracting smallpox at all. In 1796, Jenner spoke with a milkmaid called Sarah, who had contracted a much milder virus, cowpox, through milking her cow, Blossom. He collected pus from her and injected it into his test subject: James, his gardener's eight-year-old son. As predicted, James developed cowpox. Jenner then introduced the smallpox virus into young James's skin. After falling mildly ill, the boy made a full recovery.

Two years later, thanks to Jenner's work and vaccination programme, many more people were surviving smallpox in England, and the use of clinical trials to prevent disease began. The word vaccination is derived from the Latin *vacca*, meaning cow, and Blossom's hide was donated to St George's University in 1857 to commemorate Jenner's achievement. It still sits in the university library.

Henry Gray, another notable alumnus, became a medical student at St George's University in 1845. With a keen interest in human anatomy, Gray learned by dissecting each organ of the cadaver himself, instead of just watching the demonstrators carry out the dissections as his peers did.

After completing his medical studies and working as a general surgeon at St George's Hospital for a few years, Gray decided to create an anatomy textbook to share his passion for the human body with both students and surgeons alike. When he was 31, the book was first published, and later editions came to be known as *Gray's Anatomy*. Unfortunately, Gray died three years after the publication of his book, after contracting smallpox. If only Jenner's vaccination had been successful for him.

Being in the dissection room regularly made me think of John Hunter, often referred to as the father of modern surgery. Scottish-born Hunter came to London to study at St George's University in 1748, then took up a post and continued to work in the hospital as a qualified surgeon after completing his medical studies. It is said that Hunter revolutionised surgery by his insistence on observation and experimentation. He argued that all medical treatments and surgical procedures should be tried and tested first on willing subjects or cadavers, and only the therapies that worked should be introduced into practice on patients. This seems like common sense today, and slightly alarming that it wouldn't automatically have been the protocol even in the 18th century, but at the time, this type of thinking was unusual.

Like Henry Gray, Hunter also wished to pass his expertise on to others, and he did this by teaching. Unfortunately, Hunter died suddenly from a heart attack whilst in a boardroom meeting, sitting on a blue couch within the university. A heated discussion had begun about the students who were next to be enrolled into his classes, which caused a cardiac arrest and his subsequent demise. The following day, his students arrived for their usual anatomy session in the dissection room, and sat and waited for their lecturer. They soon realised, however, that he was in fact laid out on the dissecting table, his deceased cadaver awaiting the scalpel's incision.

Hunter had left prior instruction that in the event of his death, his body was to be dissected by his students, his final contribution to their learning. The fateful blue couch on which Hunter took his last breath was still on display in the foyer of St George's University during my studies.

St George's University of London specialises in healthcare and medicine, and is the only university set within a hospital in the UK. I hadn't been aware of this fact before I arrived for my course interview and was confused trying to find the university and not the hospital itself, finally realising that according to Google Maps, the two were the same thing. Thankfully, there were helpful signs and people in brightly coloured t-shirts, known as student ambassadors, at the entrance, so my confusion didn't last for too long.

On the day of my interview, after realising that I wouldn't be able to find where I needed to go by myself, I asked one of the student ambassadors, showing her a copy of my interview invitation. She kindly walked me through the hospital to the university and even rode with me up in the lift so she could show me right to the room. Regretfully, I didn't pay much attention to where she was leading me, walking blindly behind her as I rehearsed the interview answers I had prepared in my head. As a result, on the first day of the course, I was lost all over again, but this time without any student ambassadors around to help.

I had looked into and even practised the most efficient route to the university from where I had chosen to live, as well as timing it to ensure that there was no chance of me being late on the first day of the course. This journey, however, was only calculated and rehearsed to the door of the hospital, not to the lecture room within the university in which I needed to be on that first Monday morning.

The day I was due to start my course, I actually made it to the hospital ahead of time, but once inside, I realised that I had no idea where I was going and had forgotten the way. For anyone else, asking a friendly looking passer-by for directions would solve the problem, but it wasn't so easy for someone who struggled to remember directions and had difficulty differentiating their left from their right.

After walking through the hospital corridors, eventually finding the university foyer, and then the lifts, I arrived at the classroom where I needed to be, though not without the help of another kind person who took me all the way. I vowed to be as kind and helpful to any students who asked me for directions in the future, once I had learned to find my own way around the building. The comfort that came from a stranger saying 'Don't worry, I'll show you' any time directions were involved was something I both relied on and never took for granted.

I got to the classroom late, but to my relief, I wasn't the last to arrive. Nonetheless, I made a mental note to leave much earlier each morning to find the assigned lecture rooms, as they would likely change from day to day.

Walking into a classroom, especially a small one, after the lecture has started is one thing I've always dreaded. The only available seats for latecomers inevitably seem to be on the front row, preventing you from discreetly slipping in at the back, semi-invisible, no-one noticing as you get out all you need as fast as possible and pretend you have been present right from the start.

Our classroom was small, much smaller than I had expected it to be, though it was clear that we didn't need much space. We weren't a big group, after all. The room had rows of chairs facing towards the whiteboard at the front, each with a single arm rest which folded out and doubled as a small desk. Most of these armrests were on the right side of the chairs, catering to the majority of people being right-handed. I did feel sympathy for left-handed classmates who would, for the rest of the course, have to be beady eyed to spot the couple of left-sided chairs as quickly as possible to avoid having nothing to rest their elbow on as they wrote their notes.

Despite the white painted walls and large windows spanning the entire back wall, the room was still quite dark and shadowy. This was because it overlooked an adjacent hospital ward, which had its curtains closed for privacy. The university was built up over many floors, providing great views across London if you were lucky enough to be in the right room, facing the right direction. Otherwise, your view consisted of clouds and closed ward curtains.

Eventually, all the new physician associate students who were expected to attend had arrived on that first morning. We all sat with friendly but uncertain expressions on our faces, trying to assess each other and the situation that we'd voluntarily placed ourselves in: to be students, again. It was clear who would be the more confident and outspoken and who would be the quiet and reserved characters, even in the first few minutes.

We were all strangers who had been chosen, out of many applicants, to embark on this new adventure to become physician associates. Perhaps underneath it all, we felt that we had a point to prove to each other and ourselves: that we deserved to sit in the seats we currently occupied, and that the interviewers hadn't made some terrible mistake in selecting us. Although it's possible that it was only me who felt this way. As I glanced around the room, I noticed some familiar faces from my own interview day, and I was happy to see them again. There were also some faces that I had expected to see who weren't there, people who'd seemed outstanding in the group activity of the interview, but were not present in the room.

There was a good mixture of males and females, though more females. There was also a broad age range, with myself being the youngest. I had anticipated this as I had been the youngest on my undergraduate course, too, and had started this one almost straight after graduating. My classmates all came from different occupations: a nurse, a radiographer, an ophthalmologist, biomedical scientists and more. There were those who had just graduated, like myself, and those who had been working in their chosen field for a while before applying for this course. There were people of different religions and nationalities; people who were parents, married or singletons. It was a wide variety of smart strangers.

We started off as a cohort of 25. Whilst this might seem like a low number, it was actually the largest physician associate cohort to date. The course was growing more and more each year, but still only had a small intake annually – very different to today's courses with dozens of students in each cohort. My undergraduate cohort had also been small, so I was used to the dynamics of this. It meant that we'd spend a lot of time with each other as there was less need for breakout groups and seminars. We'd learn our colleagues' names more quickly, and also their bad habits, irks and irritations. We'd learn about each other's personal lives, strengths and insecurities.

There were those who needed to be heard and seen; there were those who listened and observed quietly, taking everything in. Naturally, there were people who gravitated towards each other, spending more time in the company of each other outside of the classroom, but give or take a few minor disagreements – no more than you would expect from a group of strangers working together all day, every weekday – as a whole, we got on really well as a group.

With most university courses, the first few lectures are nothing to do with your chosen subject at all and could cover topics that you might not have expected, like money management and budgeting, emotional wellbeing, fire safety etc – generic but important things for every student to know. In my first year as an undergraduate, being so keen to get going and start learning, I thought that there had been some terrible mistake when I got my first week's timetable, that I had been enrolled on to the wrong course. I soon realised that everyone's timetable looked the same as it was part of our orientation and induction, standing us in good stead for the rest of our degree.

With the physician associate course, on the other hand, no time was wasted and we jumped straight into cardiology in the first lecture. This time, I wouldn't have minded a week or two on stress management and budgeting, but every lecture counted. The human body is weird and wonderful, and we needed to learn all about it as efficiently as possible within the two-year course.

Our lecturers were a mixture of qualified physician associates and GPs who were also educators, all with their own teaching methods, standards and expectations, and we were definitely pushed hard. In the first lecture, we were told that the following week, we would have a test on medical terminology. Despite working as a healthcare assistant for the past couple of years, I didn't know any medical terminology, or at least, not the terminology that I assumed would be included in the test. I could only just about manage layman's terminology.

'I'm dyslexic and cannot learn medical terminology in a week!' I wanted to scream.

As soon as the last lecture finished on the day the test was announced, I made my way straight to the library to find the best medical terminology book available. However, I failed the test, despite studying hard for the entire week. I vowed it would be the last exam that I would fail over this full-on two-year course. But I was wrong – like most of my answers for the medical terminology exam, apparently.

For a lot of my peers, especially those who had studied anatomy or biomedical science, many things that the lecturers touched on or mentioned during the first few weeks were building on knowledge that they already had. I realised, though, that for me, all of what I was being taught was brand new information and the first time I had heard of any of these strange words, conditions and body parts. It fascinated me, but equally intimidated me. The whole point of this being a postgraduate course, with a prerequisite of health-related undergraduate learning and healthcare experience, was that we students would already have a good basis on which to build our knowledge. There was no time to start at the basic level, so a certain foundation was assumed.

Because I had majored in health studies and minored in human bioscience, there were gaps in my scientific foundation knowledge. However, for the first time since the end of primary school, being a self-professed stationery enthusiast, perhaps even hoarder, paid off. The writing, annotating, highlighting and colour coding of lecture notes was an essential skill and I was more than prepared.

The first year of the course was mainly classroom-based lectures, mixed in with small-group-style learning, dissection room practicals and half a day per week at our allotted general practice. I enjoyed the lectures, but often struggled to remember any of what had been covered five minutes after the lecture had ended and would painstakingly go through it all again in the evenings. I had always wanted to learn about the human body, to study disease and medicine, and now I was doing just that.

Lectures tended to run from 9am to 5 or 6pm, five

days a week. No half days. No half weeks. A full timetable for the full-on course. Attendance was mandatory, except in the event of a personal crisis or alien abduction. This was never a problem for me, though, as on the whole, I loved being there.

However, problem-based learning (PBL) was something I dreaded each week. The premise was that we were all given a list of questions relating to a system that we had been or were about to study. Individually, we would find the answers through textbooks and the internet, and then come together as a group to go over what we had learned. For this, the class was broken into smaller groups of about six, and each group was allocated its own room and a PBL tutor who facilitated the session, though the idea was that it was more or less led by us students.

Answering each question took me a long time throughout the week. Finding the answers themselves wasn't too difficult, as the gigantic library copies of Kumar and Clark's *Clinical Medicine* or online resources provided them. The problem for me was, after I had read through the pages and condensed the answers into my notebook, what I had just written would vanish from my memory, which is common for people with dyslexia. And it was important I knew the information well by the time of the PBL session so that I could stand in front of my highly intelligent peers and convincingly 'teach' them, looking at my notes as little as possible. If we provided too little information, the tutor would try to prise more out of us to challenge us, and this was something that I really didn't enjoy.

The way I tried to survive PBL sessions was to find the answers to all the questions, but volunteer to answer the easiest ones where possible. The downside of this was that for me, they were all equally difficult. At the end of a term, we would all give a written review of each other's contribution to the PBL group, another aspect I did not like. Basically, it felt like everyone else was a human body genius and I was just Chloe.

My colleagues were kind and supported me in the group, finishing my sentences when my mind was a blank and encouraging me with reassuring smiles, allowing me time to gather my thoughts before answering a question. The feedback they gave was always constructive, though I couldn't really apply it as I was already doing everything they suggested. Very few knew how extremely difficult certain things were for me, because I didn't want them to know. In the real world, I wouldn't be able to stand before a patient and say, 'Mrs Smith, I know what's wrong with you, but I can't explain it to you because I'm dyslexic, you see.'

I needed to find the way to make it work, no excuses, while being kind to myself too.

Ever since my acceptance email had popped into my inbox just a few months prior, informing me that I had been successful in securing a place on the course, I had thought about it daily. A 'love/hate' relationship seems too strong to describe how I felt about education and studying; a 'love/strong difficulty' relationship would be much more accurate.

I had graduated well from my undergraduate course with an upper second-class honours classification, and I was grateful for the help and support that I'd received along the way. However, there was still some doubt and uncertainty mixed in with my excitement. I'm sure that my peers experienced a not too dissimilar emotion, but my own reservations were more related to whether I had learned enough skills to minimise the effects that dyslexia and dyscalculia could have on my studies.

The words 'intensive' and 'in-depth', mentioned on the course information page, had caused me the most uncertainty. A lot of courses claim to be intensive and requiring full-time study, but really, this isn't the case. I had a feeling, though, based on the syllabus we'd need to cover in the two years of the course, in this case, the description was completely accurate.

I reminded myself that this period of study would be different from the others. I would be aware of my strengths, weaknesses and general difficulties from the very beginning. The skills and methods that I was taught during the undergraduate course, such as effective ways to study and assignment writing, were fresh in my mind. I just had to put them to the test, on paper and in real life.

Disease and sickness, despite the upheaval, disruption and sadness they cause, fascinated me far more than good health. I found that the more sinister and unusual the symptoms, the more I was engaged and able to retain the information in the lectures. The more shocking the stories, the more I could recall the details in my revision. So places like the dissection room were environments where my learning tended to be very productive, particularly if the cadavers had visible physical disease.

I remember once poking at a hard lump on the lung that I was holding and examining in a dissection room session. It was an ugly lump, ruining the aesthetic of the otherwise pleasing body part.

'Chloe, you can't poke away the cancer,' the session facilitator joked. 'It's well embedded within the cells.' I had never seen cancer before. And whilst it had been a large contributor to the patient's demise, I was still fascinated by this ugly mass nestling snugly in my cadaver's lung.

Another place that entertained my fascination with the weird and wonderful human body was the university's pathology museum. The word pathology refers to the cause and effect of disease, and the museum itself is home to a collection of thousands of human specimens with either disease or deformity. The original specimen was donated in 1843, and has been perfectly preserved since.

Despite its gruesome contents, the pathology museum reminded me of a cosy old library, with low ceilings and yellow lighting, walls covered in rows and rows of shelves. The main difference was that instead of the shelves containing hundreds of books, they contained hundreds of jars of various body parts, organs and tissue, all with a story written on a little piece of paper below. The jars were not to be picked up or held, unlike the specimens in the dissection room, only admired by the eyes. And in some of the jars, a pair of eyes would be staring right back at you.

CHAPTER 7

NEW ARRIVALS

I remember as a child contemplating my future career options, and for a short period of time, I considered training to be a midwife. This decision was solely based on the misconception that after I had delivered the babies, I would then hold, cuddle and coo over them for the rest of the day. Unless, of course, I had other babies to deliver on that shift.

After discussing this with my Aunt, who at the time was a midwife herself, and receiving the shocking revelation that my preconceptions were inaccurate, I quickly changed my mind back to pursuing a career in medicine. However, whilst on the physician associate course, I was excited to learn that one of our compulsory placements would be in obstetrics and gynaecology, or obs and gynae for short, the hospital department in which my fantasy midwifery career would have taken place.

Obs and gynae were terms that I had heard used every

now and again. I knew they related to babies somehow, but until I started studying the physician associate course, I didn't really understand much about them, nor the difference between the two terms. I soon realised that obstetricians are doctors who work alongside midwives, focusing on the mother's pregnancy and delivering babies, whilst gynaecologists are doctors who specialise in the female reproductive system such as the vagina, cervix, ovaries and nearby structures and organs. Despite the similarities, the main difference is that obstetric patients are either pregnant or have recently delivered their baby, whilst gynaecology patients vary significantly in terms of their medical concern and range from teenagers to elderly women (patients younger than teens are typically managed by paediatricians). They can present with any problem relating to the female anatomy.

My obs and gynae placement took place at Blue Hospital and the clinical supervisor that I was provided with was a warm and welcoming consultant, well known and respected in his field. As well as having physician associate and medical students to supervise, he also oversaw the development of the qualified doctors within his team who were undergoing more specialist training. Wherever my supervisor went, he seemed to have an entourage of students and doctors scuttling behind him. I saw this as confirmation of being in good hands.

As friendly as he was, he did intimidate me to begin with. This was through no fault of his own, just the natural authority he exuded without even intending to.

He was another tall consultant, well over six foot, so again I required a stool to stand on to get a clear view of the surgical procedure that he was doing. With shaved hair and bright green eyes, unusual with his caramel-coloured complexion, he was an attractive man – the type of man I would be most embarrassed about having a gynaecology appointment with.

I found out very early on that he was a supervisor who would regularly quiz his students out of the blue about patients' conditions, medications and management plans. He would start a sentence, drawing in my interest, then deliberately pause, expecting me to finish it with accurate medical information. This approach just did not work for my dyslexic brain, no matter how much I tried. In fact, it was something that I always feared.

Despite the fact that I did the recommended syllabus reading daily, being quizzed unexpectedly gave me a level of stage fright and performance anxiety that I hadn't even known I possessed. The answer, whilst on the tip of my tongue, wouldn't come into my mind. Even if I did know the answer, through fear that it might be wrong, I would say that I didn't know. This was frustrating when often, I really did.

We got on well, though. He saw through my lack of confidence and helped me to come out of my shell. On-the-spot quizzes became less regular as he tried a different approach that worked better for me, which I was extremely grateful for. We started to have more relaxed conversations about the patients and conditions we were seeing in clinics, with me scribbling down nuggets of useful information as they rolled off his tongue, and whilst I was demonstrating all the knowledge that I did have, it felt less like taking an exam I wasn't prepared for and more like a positive learning experience.

It had been a very long time since I had been to a labour ward. Years, in fact. The last time was when I had gone to meet my long-time friend Crystal's newborn daughter, Asia. Crystal had been one of the first of my friends to have a baby, providing me with a front-row-seat experience of pregnancy and motherhood.

I met Asia only moments after she'd been born. I was merely a visitor, marvelling at the beautiful newborn baby in my arms, with no responsibilities to anyone. Being on the maternity ward as a student was a very different experience.

I was with my supervisor during the day as much as possible, but for variety in my learning experience, I was placed with other consultants and clinical staff throughout my time on the placement. All of these people kindly took me under their wing.

The obstetrics and labour wards were where I was placed first. I had been given a tour of the labour ward and was definitely impressed, compared to wards in other hospitals where I had worked so far. I knew that if I was ever admitted to hospital and given a choice of ward, regardless of the ailment, I would choose a labour ward just for fun.

At Blue Hospital the labour ward was bright and calming. Each large room generally had one bed and neutral decor. The beds seemed bigger than normal, though perhaps this was because of the extra-large and bouncy pillows.

Further along the corridor was the birthing centre. This was a single spacious room with a bed, again with large fluffy pillows, brightly coloured bean bags to sit on and big, shiny yoga balls on the floor in the corner. There was a light feature along the wall, giving the entire room a soothing multicoloured glow. The artwork relaxed me as if by magic. The general ambience was enhanced by the ever-smiling midwives, students and other staff floating around the ward like angelic postmen and women, delivering babies instead of mail.

What I originally found strange was the big circular bath in the room. I was later told that this was for water births, not for a long soak and scrub as I had originally assumed. Despite the ward being the location of the most screams in the entire hospital and perhaps the whole of Borough, the atmosphere was tranquil and quiet. There must have been a lot of soundproofing within the walls.

By the ward's main doors were the locker rooms for staff to change into the blue scrubs that were provided. We were all advised to wear the scrubs to help prevent infection. There were also wipe-able rubber mules, like crocs, or plastic shoe covers for if we preferred to keep our own shoes on. However, it didn't take long for me to realise just how messy labour was, so I was grateful that my own personal clothing and shoes remained safe and clean back in the locker room next door.

The thing that I was most excited to observe on this entire placement was the delivery of a baby. I had never witnessed a baby being born before. The obstetricians floated between all the mothers in active labour, whereas the midwives had their fixed patients who they stayed with from the start of labour until the end. My obstetric supervisor for the day asked if I wanted to float with her or stay with a midwife and her patient, and I chose the latter so I could observe the entire process.

When the patient was asked if she minded my presence in the room, she graciously stated that she didn't mind at all. I wondered, if the tables were turned and I was asked if a stranger could watch me push a baby out into the world whilst they scribbled into a notebook in a corner of the room, whether I'd be as generous.

I considered my male classmates on their obs and gynae placements. Were they faced with obstacles in their shadowing experiences? Did female patients perhaps prefer them not to be in the room as they underwent intimate examinations and procedures?

I had known before the placement began that my supervisor would be a man, having shared some email correspondence with him and introduced myself, but I did believe he would be the only man in the department. Once I arrived, I realised most of the gynaecology consultants were, at the time, men. There were female consultants and registrars too, but the larger number were men.

I'm sure some female patients were like myself and incredibly shy about intimate examinations. Even the thought of exposing myself to a woman was mortifying. Patients were given a choice as to the gender of their clinician, but perhaps some didn't mind or notice whether the clinician was a man or a woman, and just saw each one as there to do their job. Which, of course, they were.

The patient who had generously agreed for me to stay and observe her delivery was a woman in her forties, present with her partner who looked around the same age. They both already had children from previous relationships who were around my age, but after starting their new relationship, they decided that they wanted a child together.

Even though the mother had given birth to two healthy children in the past, that was when she was much younger and this pregnancy was considered high risk due to her age. This meant that she had to be closely monitored throughout her pregnancy and delivery. Her contractions had started at home and as they became more frequent, she and her partner had made their way into hospital, where she was now getting herself comfortable on the pillows. She had brought an extra pillow from home with a fancy pillowcase, and her own blanket was laid across her feet. Some of her books were on her side table and a mini radio was playing soothing tunes. She looked comfortable and at home, which I was happy about, though I didn't know when she was expecting to have the time to read the books. I was excited, hoping the baby would make his or her appearance before I finished my day at 5pm.

As it turned out, things moved incredibly slowly. As the hours passed, both partners' adult children came in to visit individually, dropping off flowers and early congratulations gifts before heading away again to return later in the evening. I had been with this patient since I'd arrived at 9am, and by early afternoon, nothing else had happened.

The patient wasn't as dilated as the midwife and obstetrician had hoped, considering the time of her water breaking. Every so often, they would get out a big contraption that looked like a belt and went around the mother's protruding stomach. This was to measure the baby's heart rate and make sure he or she wasn't in distress. Thankfully, the baby wasn't, but the contractions were now much closer together and the mother, having been in pain all day, was getting exhausted before the pushing had even begun. She was visibly frustrated and worn out.

I did all I could to be helpful and not just a spectator, bringing drinks, water, cold compresses and ice, offering to heat up the warming pads that she'd brought with her, turning up and down the music as requested, helping her to reposition in the bed. It was almost as though she was there alone, but her partner remained at her side, not doing anything but being a present and quiet support.

. . .

At some point around 4pm, the midwife popped her head round the door and asked me to speak with her in the corridor. This immediately made me panic. Was I about to get into trouble? I couldn't think of anything I had done wrong as I had been nothing but attentive to my expectant mother.

It turned out the midwife had spoken to her colleague, another midwife on shift whose patient was just about ready to deliver. She was offering me the opportunity to change patients, in order to increase my chances of seeing a long-awaited delivery before the end of the day. Although I didn't like to give up on the mother I was with and felt we had come so far together, I was very keen to meet a newborn baby at this stage. I went back in to explain this to the couple, wished them the best of luck, and then went to meet my new patient.

A woman with her husband at her side, the new patient had long, dark, wavy hair and thick eyelashes that looked like extensions. She had a fresh manicure and matching pedicure. I hoped I would look as great as this woman only moments before bringing a human life into the world.

Despite being in active labour with regular contractions, she seemed genuinely pleased to meet me, asking me about myself and my studies. She even asked if I needed a chair, not that she was in any position to pop out of the room and grab me one. This was her first child and despite her waters only having broken a short while ago, the baby was ready to meet his parents.

The patient was sitting upright, propped up by her pillows. Her legs were opened wide, knees up with her feet planted firmly onto the bed. Her husband clutched on to one of her legs whilst holding her hand and gazing at her in awe.

The contractions were coming in thick and fast. Before we knew it, it was time for Mum to start doing the big pushes. Guided by the midwife, with each command to push, Mum obediently bore down and gave it her all, red in the face and holding her breath until the contraction had passed. Her husband, I noticed, was absentmindedly holding his breath too.

I was positioned at the side of the patient's bed and wanted to look down at what was happening. Normally, out of respect for other people's privacy, I would avoid looking at the intimate areas of a patient unless I had received explicit consent. I didn't want to assume that because this patient had allowed me to be in the room during her labour, she also didn't mind me staring into her vagina. It definitely wasn't the appropriate time to ask for clarification.

Almost as though she could see into my mind and read my thoughts, in between puffs and pants, she whispered, 'It's OK, you can look, don't be shy.' I wasn't shy, but I was worried that another pair of eyes focused on her genitals would make *her* feel shy. I was clearly wrong.

I looked down. At first, I couldn't decipher quite what

I was looking at. I'd never seen a baby's head crowning before, but I hadn't expected it to look like this.

I could see a small area of the top of the baby's head, only a few centimetres, and his dark hair. The skin appeared to be a whitish-greyish colour, and his head was the most peculiar shape. Not round, that's for sure. I expected the midwife to vocalise a version of my own alarm, but instead, she smiled and told Mum that she was doing great, she could see the head and Mum was nearly there.

The atmosphere was tense. I was convinced that the baby was extremely deformed and the midwife had not yet realised it, and that she, Mum and Dad would be in for a terrible shock once he was delivered. In the background, almost drowned out by the grunts, shouts and panting, relaxing, soothing tunes, similar to those playing to my first patient, reminded me of the music I would expect to hear in a spa – an environment so different to our current one.

Mum was informed that with the next contraction, she was to give the biggest push that she could manage, which would likely be her last before labour was over. The contraction started and Mum took a big inhale and squeezed her husband's hand until the skin on both their knuckles went white. Beads of sweat ran off her forehead and gathered in the furrows of her frowning eyebrows before running down her face like tears.

With a roar of triumph from Mum, the baby's head emerged fully, gently guided by the midwife. The rest of his body and all four little limbs followed and nestled into the midwife's towel-covered hands.

Whilst it was emerging, the baby's head had resembled a rugby ball, not the perfectly rounded football that I had expected. By the time he was cleaned and placed naked on to Mum's chest, his head seemed to have rounded itself. I was later reassured that the baby's head was completely normal. The shape that had so alarmed me was the result of his skull being soft enough to flex and help with delivery. As he grew, his skull would harden.

Mum was in tears, Dad was in tears, the newborn baby boy was most definitely in tears. I too blinked back some tears of my own. While Mum and Dad cuddled up, cradling their new baby, the midwife was still busy, cutting, clamping, delivering, wiping and stitching away. Mum in particular seemed oblivious to everything going on around her, almost in a trance-like state of love with the tiny human on her chest who she had waited so long to meet.

It was well past time for me to go home, but I'd had a wonderful day, witnessing the miracle of childbirth through the generosity of the shared experiences with both of the super-mums. I thanked the new parents I was with and slipped out of the room as they posed for selfies. Childbirth was simply beautiful, but if I was honest, it wasn't as glamorous as I had thought it was going to be. As far as I could remember, on *Friends*, Rachel giving birth to Emma didn't seem to involve so many different bodily fluids and solids.

On my way out of the ward, I found the original midwife, the one who had realised how keen I was to see a birth and arranged for it to happen, and asked how her mother was getting on. The baby had turned out to be breach, meaning she was lying in the wrong position, which was why Mum had not been progressing further into labour as expected. Mum had been wheeled off to surgery to have a caesarean section, and now both she and her baby girl were doing well.

I changed my clothes in the changing room and left the ward to head home, questioning whether I would have what it takes to push a whole baby out into the world. Despite it being the 21st century – a century full of groundbreaking new medical advances – childbirth still has its risks. There are incidents of physical trauma, injury, and even death for mother, baby and sometimes both. In the UK, these risks are significantly higher for mothers from ethnic minorities, particularly black mothers, who are four times more likely to die in childbirth than Caucasian mothers. And whilst studies and reports, along with public petitions, have called for urgent action across the country to address this scary disparity in maternal outcome, there is still a long way to go to close the gap in health inequality.

In the corridor ahead of me, walking towards me, was a man. I recognised him to be the expectant dad I had been with earlier that day, the one whose partner had just undergone surgery to deliver their baby safely. And he appeared to recognise me too, despite me wearing completely different clothes to the light blue scrubs he had last seen me in. I smiled and went to say goodbye to him, but he signalled for me to hold on a moment, putting up a single finger.

I stood in front of him with a puzzled and nervous smile on my face as he fished around in his jeans pocket. I was hoping that he wasn't going to offer me money. As a student, I found cash a welcome, and frequent, gift from my own family, but it was highly inappropriate from a patient, or their partner.

He handed me a small piece of paper and said, 'Here, I wrote down my number for you earlier, but then you left and I didn't see you for the rest of the afternoon. Give me a call sometime.' Then he winked and walked off, back to his partner, who was waiting for him on the ward while recovering from emergency surgery, and their newborn daughter.

I stood on the spot for a little while, astounded and angry. Perhaps I had misheard him or misunderstood what had just happened. But as I continued to walk out of the hospital and towards my bus stop, I realised that I hadn't misunderstood. That new dad had definitely just hit on me.

I felt devastated. Not for me, but for his partner and baby. Part of me kicked myself for not telling him off there and then, rather than just standing silent, wide mouthed and even wider eyed. Part of me wanted to go back and tell her what he had just done. But I didn't. Instead, I threw his number into a bin I passed on the street, hoping never to see him again.

A disappointing ending to a beautiful day.

A caesarean or C-section was something else that I was looking forward to seeing for the first time. This is the surgical method of delivering the baby by making an incision through the lower abdomen and the uterus. With a vaginal delivery, even after the mother's water breaks, the baby arrives when it chooses to arrive, and until it does, everyone has to wait patiently. With a C-section, things move along much more quickly.

When the C-section is elective, it means that it is planned during the pregnancy, and the mother and her obstetrician choose the exact date that she will have the surgery to deliver the baby. An emergency C-section happens when a vaginal delivery was the original plan, but due to complications or changes in circumstances or health, it is no longer the best option and the mother is taken to surgery.

I was shadowing a friendly obstetrician who was as excited as I was that this would be my first time seeing the C-section procedure. She let me scrub in, which means that I prepped myself for surgery, washing my hands and arms meticulously before the scrub team helped me to put on my long sterile gown, gloves, mask and face shield. I didn't understand the need for the face shield initially and was concerned it would obstruct my view. Not much later on, I was extremely grateful for it.

The mother was already prepped for the surgery and lying on the bed by the time the consultant and I entered the operating theatre with our hands out in front us, careful not to touch a single thing. What startled me slightly was the amount of people inside the operating theatre. I had expected it just to be the mother, father, myself and the consultant. On top of that was an anaesthetist sitting at one side of the mother, monitoring different screens and the patient's observations. There were people responsible for other tasks too, but I didn't catch it all, despite everything being explained to me. I was too excited.

The patient had just had an epidural, a type of numbing procedure that would prevent her from feeling anything from the waist downwards. She had a handy curtain across the top of her stomach, separating the two halves of her body so she wouldn't be able to see herself being cut open. There were midwives at the head end of the patient, talking to her, asking her questions, helping to make her feel comfortable. On the stomach side of the curtain, where I stood, there were staff responsible for handing the obstetrician the correct instruments when they were needed.

Once the surgery started and the first incision was made, I braced myself for the mother to cry out in pain, but I could hear her and her husband calmly discussing baby names. Although I couldn't see her face behind the curtain, she was clearly unable to feel the scalpel's lacerations, chiselling away at her stroke by stroke.

The procedure wasn't as bloody as I had expected it to be, as one of the members of the team was responsible for holding a mini vacuum device, which sucked up the blood in order to keep the obstetrician's view unobstructed. It was so critically important that she could see clearly throughout the procedure. As the incision cut across the lower part of the mother's stomach, through tissue, muscle and fat, I was surprised by just how deep it went. I expected the obstetrician to reach the mattress at any moment.

After she'd cut through the uterus, the amniotic sac was clearly visible and a wonder to behold. It resembled a giant water balloon with a small live human inside, rolled up into a ball and wriggling around slowly. The final incision was a little nick against the taut membrane of the amniotic sac, which caused a gush of fluid to drain onto the nearby towels and dressings already in place. The fluid shot out with such force that I was grateful for the face shield, even though it did not reach me as I was now standing at the foot of the bed.

The baby girl was retrieved, the umbilical cord was cut. After a brief wipe down with a towel, the baby was taken round to the other side of the curtain to meet her parents, whilst the mother's abdominal cavity was sutured back together carefully, layer by layer.

· · ·

Aside from watching new life being bought into the world, there was so much more to see within the obs and gynae specialty. My timetable was varied and packed with different sorts of clinics, surgeries and procedures, most onsite at the hospital and one a short bus ride away at an offsite gynae clinic.

One afternoon, I was invited by one of the registrars to sit in on her pessary clinic. I had been working with this registrar, but I wasn't yet scheduled to see such a clinic, so I had no idea even what a pessary was. Nonetheless, I was grateful for the invitation and I went along.

Sometimes, in older women and those who have given birth to multiple children, the vaginal walls are not as strong as they used to be and don't stay up on their own, causing a collapse, or a prolapse to use the correct terminology. I soon discovered that vaginal pessaries are firm plastic rings that are inserted into the vagina. They sit at the top, working almost as scaffolding, keeping the vaginal walls and other structures up and in place, preventing a prolapse. In the pessary clinic, the patient would lie on the bed and the gynaecologist would simply remove the old pessary and replace it with a new one.

Pessaries come in different sizes, meaning the vagina has to be measured before one is fitted and inserted. It's then changed every six months or so, which is an extremely intimate procedure. I was impressed by how little the female patients seemed bothered by it all, often making small talk with me as I stood and observed, and wishing me well with my studies.

The colposcopy clinic was another part of my obs and gynae placement. This was carried out in a surgical setting similar to that for a C-section, though it was more of a procedure than full surgery, so it tended to take less time. This meant the patient would be able to go back home the same day, and that there wasn't the need for so many people in the room.

After a woman has had a routine smear, if the results suggest cervical cell changes, this needs to be examined more closely, which takes place in the colposcopy clinic. The procedure is done by using a tiny camera attached to an instrument that goes inside the vagina and up to the cervix to either cauterise and gently burn the abnormal cells, or cut away a thin layer of cells and remove them. The cells that are removed are sent to the lab to be examined closely under a microscope in order to determine whether they are OK and just need to be monitored, or more intervention is required.

The camera on the instrument transmits live footage on to the screen in the theatre, meaning that I was able to see what the consultant was seeing and doing. It felt as though I was doing the procedure myself, but I was so glad that I wasn't. There was no room for error, a tremble of hand or a lapse of concentration.

I had expected to learn a lot on my obs and gynae placement, but not as much as I actually did. Where I'd thought I understood the female body, I realised that this had just been the tip of a very large iceberg. I didn't realise how adaptable and fascinating it is, especially through pregnancy and labour, and how after delivery, the body usually changes back, physically, hormonally and structurally, to how it was before pregnancy. There were points on the placement where I felt like women in general had been served the raw end of the deal in relation to their anatomy and biology, and the potential problems that went along with them – trying to conceive, being pregnant, vaginal labour, C-sections, vaginal surgical procedures, pelvic problems, growths, tumours, cysts, period disorders, intimate examinations, urinary infections, bladder problems, incontinence, prolapses and so much more. But the more I learned and observed, the more I began to appreciate just how strong and magnificent the female body is, and I feel truly grateful to have one of my own.

CHAPTER 8

SMALL SOLDIERS

'Do you like *Dora the Explorer*, Chloe?' the paediatrician asked me with a smile on her face.

'She's OK, I guess, though not usually my TV programme of choice,' I answered, confused and amused in equal measures.

'Why don't you go and watch an episode with that patient? The ward is quiet, and if I need you for anything, I can come get you.' The paediatrician was looking at the little girl in the bed in front of us.

'Absolutely,' I answered hesitantly, unsure if this was a strange test I was being put through to see if I would pass or fail.

'It's better that she doesn't get herself too upset because we need her pulse and oxygen to stay at a nice, steady level,' the paediatrician explained. 'Her parents asked if there was anyone who could sit with her for a little while and I had you in mind.'

'Well, in that case, I'd be honoured!' I said.

The patient's parents, who had two other children, had both needed to leave the ward for a little while, but her mother was coming back in an hour. Goodbyes are always difficult for any three-year-old, let alone an unwell three-year-old by herself in a hospital bed on a paediatric intensive care unit (PICU).

At the time, the little girl was watching cartoons on the iPad provided by the ward. This iPad came in a bright, bulky wipe-able case in the shape of a pink elephant. She was sitting upright, propped up by pillows, and in front of her on the table across her bed was a beaker of juice, a pink crazy straw already positioned close to her mouth so when she wanted a sip, she didn't have to move more than a centimetre. The scene reminded me of a spa, and all she needed was a white robe, towelling turban on her head and sliced cucumbers over her eyes to complete the ensemble.

Whilst her parents tried to coordinate and alternate their time between their daughter on the ward and their other children, one of whom was a young baby, today, something unexpected had come up and both had to leave at the same time. They explained to her as well as they could, showered her with hugs and kisses, promising to be back soon, but still, their daughter cried for them to return. It broke my heart, and it must have shown on my face, hence the paediatrician I was working with nominating me for *Dora the Explorer* duties.

I put on a disposable gown and gloves – required for

all close contact with patients, even if I would not be administering medical care – and went and sat in the freshly cleaned chair next to the bed where the little girl's mother had been just moments before. I introduced myself and asked if I could sit with her and watch what she was watching.

Her eyes lit up as she told me she was watching *Dora the Explorer*. She introduced me to each of the teddies on her bed, and asked if I had any teddies of my own. After I'd explained that I didn't, she was adamant that I was to take one of hers home with me to sleep with that night.

I was blown away by how bright and confident this little girl was. She had an amazing vocabulary and entertaining sense of humour. She asked me if I knew *Doc McStuffins*, because I 'looked like her'. This made my day, as I *did* know who Doc Mcstuffins was: an animated seven-year-old black doctor from the TV programme of the same name, who had a magical pink stethoscope – the same colour as my own. Doc Mcstuffins was best friends with a lamb, dinosaur, fish, hippo and snowman, each of whom would be unwell in turn, and the magic pink stethoscope would help them get better.

I told the little girl that I didn't know Doc Mcstuffins personally, but was a huge fan of her work. We went on to watch an episode of *Dora the Explorer* and by the time it had finished, she was fast asleep. I lowered her bed a little with the remote control, switched off the iPad to preserve the battery and rejoined the paediatrician I was shadowing that day in the PICU as part of my paediatrics placement.

The PICU provides the highest level of medical treatment for unwell children, who could be brought in for many different reasons. The neonatal intensive care unit (NICU), which is similar, covers newborns. I was a little apprehensive about the time I would be spending on these units. I knew the children would be extremely unwell and was worried I would be a mere spectator of a parent's worst nightmare, unable to do much other than watch.

The PICU and NICU differ from the main paediatrics ward as they are smaller and have fewer beds, though a similar amount of staff. This means that there is a higher ratio of staff to patients, for the increased medical needs that the patients have.

My little *Dora the Explorer* patient seemed a lot more medically well than the other children on the ward, so I asked the doctor why she was there. Apparently, she'd had a severe asthma attack a couple of days before, and whilst she had made a speedy recovery with the help of oxygen, adrenaline and steroids, she was still under observation due to how quickly she had originally deteriorated. The team was watchful, but no longer worried about her. Her observations remained stable and things were looking positive for her to be discharged soon. I was glad that she'd recovered well, and hoped that she would be back home with her family and teddies in no time.

Paediatrics as a specialty focuses solely on the medical care of children from birth up to the age of 16 and, under certain circumstances, up to 18. The Orange Hospital that I was doing my paediatric placement at was close to the university. Amongst all the clinical students, clinical placements at Orange Hospital were always coveted and everyone wanted them.

Whilst Orange Hospital was indeed a good hospital, I couldn't help but wonder if the high demand was merely to do with its close proximity to our student accommodation. As with many student experiences, the majority of us had moved away from home into accommodation closer to the university, either in the halls of residence or private renting with other students nearby. With being expected to attend a placement from early in the morning until the evening, we regarded a hospital that was close to home as the ultimate luxury. It was the simple things that brought us the most pleasure as students.

Initially, when our individual placement timetables were given to us, I was a little disappointed by how many different hospitals I would have to attend. I had hoped that all of my placements for the course would be at St George's Hospital, even though I had been told early on that the locations would vary. As it transpired, only four out of my ten placements were at St George's.

By the end of the rotations, I was grateful to have experienced and worked in so many hospitals and environments, despite my initial apprehension. At this stage in my life, a lot of my decisions revolved around what my dyslexia would allow me to do comfortably with minimal stress. Travelling to new places was my biggest fear, but without doing that very thing, how was I ever to improve?

My paediatric supervisor was a well-known and very accomplished clinician in her field. She was also the co-author of the clinical handbook that I was currently using for my revision, which I found extremely impressive. She was young, but considering how experienced she was, I guess she was likely older than she looked. Friendly and warm, she encouraged conversation and the asking of questions. She wore her blonde hair in a short bob and had a kind face, one that I'm sure her young patients would have appreciated.

The main paediatric ward, similar to the delivery ward, radiated calm and peacefulness. Even though some of the children were extremely unwell and their parents, sitting at their bedsides, were understandably anxious, the environment clearly tried its best to cater to children as much as it could. Famous cartoon characters decorated the walls and corridors, and the ward had its own playroom kitted out with a TV and a table providing ample sheets of blank paper, pictures to be coloured in and felt tips and crayons all the colours of the rainbow, allowing for young artists' creations to come to life. There were iPads, the furniture was mini-sized, and the staff were dedicated to encouraging and facilitating the children to play with each other each day.

One thing that my supervisor told me early on was that on the paediatrics ward, we wouldn't just have to look after the young patients, but their parents too. I soon began to understand what she meant. Not being a parent myself, initially, I struggled to appreciate how scary it must be to have an unwell child, especially one so sick they need to stay in hospital. For all good parents, it's their heart's desire to keep their child safe from harm, happy and healthy at all times. Unfortunately, there often isn't anything that a parent can do to prevent illness and accidents. All they can do is be there to support and comfort their child.

Growing up in Wellingborough, I'd had a few pet rabbits, but my favourite was my last rabbit, called Ruby. Ruby was a fluffy grey lop-eared rabbit I'd had since he was a baby. We were originally told he was a girl, but when he impregnated his female sibling, we realised the error. By this time, I felt it was too late to change his name, so Ruby he remained.

Ruby reminded me of a puppy. Inquisitive and active, he loved company and meeting new people. He had free rein in our large, secure back garden during the day, but would be ushered back into his hutch each night to sleep. The next morning, he would be let back out again. Our garden had so many hiding places that looking out of the window, I often wouldn't see Ruby at all, but as soon as he heard the back door or the garden gate open, he would appear at my feet, keen to welcome his human guest into his outside space. He would then follow me around, hopping and skipping as if performing just for me, but he had no concept of personal space boundaries, often sitting on my feet if I stood still for long enough.

One winter, Ruby sneezed. I thought I was imagining it until he did it again. As I looked more closely at his face, I noticed that his eyes had a glisten to them, as though he was about to shed a tear. There was no hesitation: we had to take him to the vet, who diagnosed him with a cold. I hadn't even known rabbits could get a cold!

That night, I was lying in bed, thinking about Ruby and his rabbit cold, worrying about him. I sneaked out of my bed, grabbed my phone and slipped out into the back garden to visit him, using my phone screen as a torch. I opened the hutch door and shone my phone in his face to get a clear view of whether he seemed OK or not. In truth, he seemed irritated that I had disturbed his sleep by pointing a bright light into his face.

Once I felt confident that he was indeed OK, I went back to bed. However, I repeated my midnight check on other nights over the week, until Ruby's sneezing eventually stopped and his eyes went back to their usual mischievous gleam. But it was only when I felt confident he was over the worst of it that I could stop worrying and once again have a peaceful, undisturbed night's sleep.

Of course, a pet rabbit with a cold does not even come close in comparison to a seriously ill child, but it was the closest I'd ever experienced to parents' anguish. And that was hard enough to deal with.

. . .

The patients on the paediatric wards had often been admitted through A&E and needed to spend more time in hospital as they recovered. Their parents had to put their complete trust in strangers and hope that we would do what we could for their child. This, of course, often led to parental angst, which would present in different ways towards the staff, sometimes via anger, frustration, sarcasm, desperation, silence and tears. But it was always understandable, and the longer I spent in the paediatric department over the course of the three-week placement, the better I understood.

Ward rounds in paediatrics, like on the adult medical wards, started early each morning. I had become used to ward rounds and understood them much better since my AMU placement. The structure and purpose remained the same, which meant the consultants and other staff members would do a check in with each patient one by one, assessing and discussing how their health was doing along with treatment plans for the day.

The main difference on the paediatric ward was that the patients were often too young to express themselves, explain their symptoms and understand their treatment. Instead, where possible, the parents would provide insight, as would the nurses and the rest of the healthcare team involved with the patient's care over the past 24 hours. Patient observations like temperature, pulse, oxygen levels, whether they had eaten or gone to the toilet, whether they wanted to play and how they'd slept were important factors. A child who didn't want to play, even with their favourite toy from home, was a child who wasn't well at all.

Another thing I learned early in my paediatric placement was that children's health can be quite unpredictable. An accident at home could seem severe and the parents would worry that the child was seriously injured, potentially even life-threateningly so, but in the end, they only needed a few stitches and a cold compress. On the other hand, a child who appeared to be slightly under the weather with nothing more than a mild cold could deteriorate quickly and unexpectedly and require urgent hospital admission. These vast differences, I'm sure, made it extremely difficult for parents to know which situations could be managed at home, with a dose of Calpol and some bed rest, and which needed emergency medical attention. In paediatrics, we didn't expect parents to be trained medical professionals and would always encourage them to ask for advice if they were unsure, either by using the NHS 111 helpline, the GP, the pharmacist or, if they deemed it necessary, attending A&E.

On one particular morning, after the ward round had finished, I was introduced to my supervisor for the day, then given the opportunity to speak with one of the parents, practise my history taking and find out what had led to her child's hospital admission. This also gave me the opportunity to speak to her little boy who had already challenged me to a game of peek-a-boo while I was observing the ward round. Whenever I made eye contact with him, he would hide his face with his hands and giggle.

I walked over to where the mum was reading at her son's bedside, introduced myself and asked if she was happy for me to speak with her. Her son, who she introduced as Nathaniel, listened eagerly, seemingly proud that he had been specially selected. Nathaniel had an enviable amount of energy for such an early hour of the morning and I could tell that he was likely feeling much better than when he had first been admitted on to the ward. He had a cute round face with big brown eyes, one of which was almost completely swollen shut.

Nathaniel's mum explained that she had noticed a tiny pimple on his top eyelid that looked like a simple stye and decided to monitor it. Over the next couple of days, the entire top and bottom of the eyelid had continued to swell, along with the side of his face. Nathaniel had started to complain that his eye hurt. Then he got a high fever and wouldn't eat even his favourite meals, which was when his mum brought him to A&E.

Nathaniel was diagnosed with periorbital cellulitis, a skin infection around the eye. He was admitted on to a ward and treatment with intravenous antibiotics and fluids started right away. The doctors looking after him were concerned that without swift intervention, the infection would progress and could potentially permanently affect his eye and eyesight.

Mum had spent the night with Nathaniel and looked tired. Nathaniel, on the other hand, had the demeanour of someone staying at Disney World. The ward was quiet, meaning that he had all the toys, entertainment and attention of the staff at his disposal, and he knew how to capitalise on it.

After speaking with his mum and making a note in my notebook of things to revise when I got home, I was invited by Nathaniel to do some colouring with him. Sadly, I had to decline his invitation as I needed to do some work.

I'm happy to say that Nathaniel responded well to his hospital treatment. Over the next few days, the symptoms completely cleared and he was discharged home.

Another patient I was able to speak to was a teenager called Rebecca, who was in hospital suffering a sickle cell crisis. Sickle cell disease is a result of abnormally shaped red blood cells, and is most commonly seen in people from African and Caribbean backgrounds. The red blood cells' normal shape resembles a doughnut, but in people with sickle cell disease, they are shaped more like a crescent moon or banana. To be born with sickle cell, a child has to inherit a copy of the gene from each parent, who would both be carriers, even though they don't have the disease themselves.

The abnormally shaped blood cells often don't live as long as normal ones, dying before the body can produce new cells, resulting in anaemia. Sickle cell anaemia causes sufferers to become tired and prone to infections, sometimes delays puberty and growth, and can even affect vision. Generally, these patients are managed at home with the input of haematologists – doctors who specialise in blood.

Ideally, once a paediatric patient is treated, their illness or injury is completely resolved and they are discharged home with no further need to return to hospital. For patients like Rebecca, this sadly is not the case. Her condition required admissions into hospital over and over again.

There are different types of sickle cell crises, but the most common is called vaso-occlusive. This happens when the abnormally shaped red blood cells get stuck and cause a blockage in the blood vessel, instead of moving freely and delivering oxygen to the rest of the body. Because the oxygen within the sickled blood cell does not arrive at the tissue that needs it, the tissue dies.

These blockages can happen in any of the blood vessels anywhere in the body, and are extremely painful and traumatic for the patient. The crisis typically lasts about a week, during which the patient has to receive very strong pain relief in the hospital, and sometimes oxygen to help them breathe.

Rebecca had been in hospital for a few days by the time I met her, being treated by all the paediatricians on the ward and the haematologists. She was coming to the end of a particularly bad sickle cell crisis, and although she was in discomfort and still not well, she was in good spirits and happy to talk to me and allow me to practise my history taking skills. Rebecca told me about what had happened, her experiences and how sickle cell affected her daily life. It was a very sad story, yet her optimism and general resilience humbled and inspired me.

Rebecca taught me a lot about sickle cell disease and even drew useful diagrams, which I kept and later used for exam revision. It was interesting for me to see this teen so mature and grounded, despite suffering with a debilitating disease that has no cure, resulting in her regularly needing to be admitted into hospital. She was so different from the teenagers that I was looking after in my part-time evening job, which I had taken on to boost my funds whilst studying.

In the second year of my course, I applied to be a resident advisor (RA) at the university's halls of residence. This job involved me working in a team with six other postgraduate students, and each evening, we would take it in turns to be on call throughout the night and hold the RA phone. By this time, I lived in the halls of residence, as did my six RA colleagues. Thankfully, we were allowed to go to sleep during our shift, but had to make sure to answer the phone promptly, meaning that we set it to the loudest, most annoying ringtone and the strongest vibration, just to be on the safe side.

The role of the RA was to provide holistic overnight support to any student living on campus. We also received calls from the halls of residence security guards who might need help with a drunken student who had forgotten which room they lived in, or had lost their keys on a night out. There was no cash payment for this job, but the remuneration included free accommodation in the halls of residence for the year, which was a godsend. When I moved out of Laura's house into my new accommodation, I immediately basked in the luxury of having my own en suite bathroom, something I hadn't experienced before.

Thankfully, throughout the whole time I worked in the RA role, my only calls were to help inebriated students back to their rooms without them waking up the entire student population. Most times, I didn't get any calls at all, allowing me to have a peaceful night's sleep, and awake rested and refreshed for placement the next morning.

When I did get calls, I sometimes felt like a glorified babysitter to adult-sized children, which really contrasted with the paediatric patients I was working with during the daytime. In some ways, my daytime work likely made me less tolerant to a drunken 18-year-old sobbing about being dumped by her boyfriend as I walked her back to her room.

'Well, at least you haven't had to drop out of university because you have leukaemia like the patient I was helping to look after today, who is now fighting for her life!' It sometimes took all my strength of will not to respond in this way, but that would have been neither professional nor fair. We physician associate students were all getting good at compartmentalising the things that we were hearing and seeing on our clinical placements, even though some were shocking, terrifying and sad. But we couldn't let them change the people we were, except to make sure that they helped us to become better clinicians in the not-so-distant future.

In the NICU, as all the patients on the ward were newborn babies, there were no beds, just cots and incubators. Each space occupied a comfortable chair with a new mother, father or close family member, but there were lots of factors that meant sometimes, a baby would be in the NICU by themselves for prolonged periods of time. This generally happened if the mum was too unwell herself to leave her own ward, or the dad was having to split his time between Mum and Baby, or Mum or Dad were both unavailable and their extended families were not local. This meant that most of the interaction and stimulation these newborns would get during their stay would be from the ward staff.

One day during my time on the NICU, I was asked if I would like to cuddle one of the babies, who was due to have no visitors that day. There has been lots of scientific research published looking into the benefits to newborn babies being held and cuddled, and I had recently been reading some of it. The benefits for the baby, according to the researchers' findings, include reduced stress and heart rate, increased quality of rest and sleep, and better autonomic functions. I was grateful to be of service.

The length of time each baby would need to stay on the NICU varied, dependent on their health and improvement. Some were on the unit only for a few days whereas others might stay for weeks or even months. This meant that despite all the babies being admitted as newborns, their age, size and stage of development differed dramatically, as did their health and the level of medical intervention they required.

The baby I was being asked to hold and cuddle was a premature little boy. Although tiny in size and weight, he was making his family and the clinicians proud by the speed of his growth. After cleaning my hands and putting on a gown and gloves, I was directed to sit in an armchair as the nurse temporarily removed the monitoring device from his tiny toe, and then he was placed into my eager arms. I was conscious of the cold rustling plastic of my disposable gown across the front of my body where he lay in the crease of my bent arm, so I ensured I made a barrier of blanket between that and his warm, soft skin.

He was adorable, as small as a doll, long eyelashes fluttering out from his closed eyelids and the occasional contented wiggle of his tiny pink lips. His arms and legs seemed to move independently of his body, jerking at will. I was in my element and happy to stay like this for the rest of the day.

While I cuddled the baby, I talked to the nurse about his progress so far and she explained how he was ready to be discharged from the NICU, but was just waiting for the consultant's final review. As the nurse and I spoke and the baby continued to sleep and wriggle in my arms, we hadn't noticed his dad walk on to the ward.

'Hope he's not giving you too much trouble,' Dad said quietly to me, with the wide, proud smile of a brand-new parent. He thanked me for giving his baby son cuddles in his absence, and I in return thanked him for his absence that had led to the opportunity for me to enjoy a cuddle. Dad washed his hands, and then we carefully did a swap, with me sliding the baby into his father's arms. The baby didn't stir, content to sleep peacefully wherever he lay.

My paediatrics placement allowed me the opportunity to interact with children, play games, and be silly, whilst still learning all the clinical information I needed. But paediatrics wasn't all fun and games. At times, it was scary, and at others incredibly sad. There were tragedies, losses and heartbreak, and the paediatricians I worked with seemed to have a superhuman ability to take it all in their stride, even when they didn't know whether their little patients were going to make it through the day or night.

There were patients I had said goodbye to on leaving in the evening. They'd waved back cheerfully, but by the next morning when I went to see them, their bed space was empty as they had passed away in the night. There were babies who never got to sleep in their brand-new cots waiting for them at home, siblings who had to say goodbye to each other forever, and parents' lives that were irreparably shattered.

One patient on the paediatric ward, a little boy, sat in his bed in a side room with a woman at his bedside. She was very formally dressed as she read through some documentation that she had in her hand. The conversation between the woman and the patient seemed cordial, but as I watched through the glass window, it was clear from their interactions that she wasn't his mother. In fact, this was confirmed soon afterwards by the amount of time he spent crying for his mother to come and take him home.

Then the police arrived on the ward and spoke with the doctors looking after him. When the officers had left again, I asked my supervisor what was going on and she replied that this was a case of non-accident injury – in other words, abuse. The staff in A&E who'd first seen the patient had determined that his injuries and bruises, some very old, did not match up with the story the mother was telling of how he had sustained them. Sadly, the patient confirmed the staff's fears when he was asked what had happened without his mother being present.

After the patient was admitted to the ward, neither his mother nor his father was permitted to visit him whilst the investigation took place. The lady at his bedside was his new social worker. It was terribly sad, but once the little boy's injuries were treated, he didn't return to his parents' home. His younger sister was also removed from the family home, and they were sent to be fostered together.

Paediatrics had been a career option that I had considered while I was still planning to apply to medical school. However, this placement helped to confirm that despite my love for children, paediatrics wasn't the specialty for me. By pursuing my newfound desire to work in a GP practice, I would still be seeing more than enough children to keep me happy, and I was looking forward to that.

Chapter 9

Skin Deep

I have always considered myself a lover, not a fighter, disliking confrontation and preferring a calm and friendly discussion to sort any issue. The only physical fight that I can ever remember having in my entire life was a silly altercation with one of my younger brothers before school one morning. I was around ten, so he would have been nine.

Dad had gone off to work hours before, and Mum had only just wished us goodbye. As usual, we were to walk ourselves to school next door about 15 minutes after her departure, meaning that for the time being, we were home alone. The squabble likely started over something incredibly silly and irrelevant, but we took it upon ourselves to settle the matter physically. Pushes, punches, slaps and I think a few kicks came from both sides, but after a plant was fatally injured, its broken stem causing it to droop over, we immediately called a truce and went off to school – separately, to avoid a rematch on the way.

The thing I disliked the most about the altercation was that although I gave as good as I got, and arguably even more, I came out looking much, much worse due to a skin condition I'd had for my whole life. It was strange and unlike anything I had seen on anyone else, although one of my brothers did seem to have something similar for a couple of years. However, his was very mild, and eventually he just grew out of it. Mine, on the other hand, seemed to be getting worse the older I got.

The symptoms were triggered by physical contact. It could be from scratching an itch, a brush of my cheek, a rub of my skin – the smallest and lightest touch of my body, anywhere from head to toe, could be enough to cause a reaction. The area that was touched would swell and develop hives, as some call it.

The site of the swelling generally matched the shape of the contact that had been applied. For example, if I scratched my arm with my fingernail, it would result in fingernail-shaped swellings on my skin. An inevitable brush of my clothes across my skin whilst I was getting dressed would result in mild and vague swellings across my body. Sometimes in primary school when I was bored, I would become a living canvas, doodling different images and patterns on to my skin with my nail, watching the intricate shapes swell up. My friends found it cool and my cousins found it entertaining, flicking me randomly to see what would appear on my skin a moment later.

I remember once stepping on the end of a pen at home whilst only wearing my socks on my feet. My concern wasn't breaking the pen (which I didn't) or ink leaking onto the carpet (which it didn't), but how my skin might punish me for my carelessness. Not long after I had moved the item to a more sensible place, I could feel, even without touching the area, that the sole of my foot had started to swell into the shape of the pen. And whilst I knew it wasn't a problem and wouldn't last long until the swelling under my foot went down, for a while, every step I took felt as though I was repeatedly standing on the tip of a pen.

My skin condition never bothered me, but I was always conscious that it might alarm those around me. In the past, I've had people offer to take me to A&E after I've rubbed my eye and made it swell excessively, so much so that it was nearly swollen shut. I've had people ask me if I should administer my EpiPen, looking horrified when I've told them that I don't carry one. I knew my strange skin behaviour must have a name and diagnosis, but I'd never got around to pursuing it. In any case, the symptoms literally only lasted for minutes before being gone without a trace.

On my dermatology placement, I was shadowing one of the dermatologists in his allergy clinic, sitting in the corner of the room with my notebook and pen. I had recently developed a habit of using the end of the pen lid to make dots across the back of my hand, knowing that soon the visible marks would form in the pattern that I had arranged, which changed depending on my mood.

One particular day, I was feeling a little overwhelmed with the amount of work that was piling up for me to do in the evenings: assignments, personal revision, exam prep, which I liked to start as early as possible. My mind was busy, and so was my hand as it dotted my skin.

A patient had arrived and was in the reception area, waiting to see the dermatologist. I volunteered to collect the patient's notes from outside the door, and then I handed them to the consultant. As I did so, a piece of paper fell out on to the floor, so I swooped down, picked it up and handed it over, too.

'My, my, what have we here?' the consultant said. Without following his eyeline, I assumed he had found something interesting in the patient's notes. But no, he was actually looking at my spotty hand.

'Oh, it's nothing,' I said dismissively. 'I was just poking myself with a pen and this happened. I'm fine. It doesn't hurt and will be gone in a few minutes. I have strange skin.' I hurried my words out, embarrassed, trying to both reassure the dermatologist and change the topic of conversation as quickly as possible.

'May I?' he asked. Taking my hand in his, he began to touch the individual swellings one by one. 'What marvellous dermatographia you have. I don't normally see it this pronounced. What medication have you been advised to take by your dermatologist?'

'Pardon, what did you call it? And I don't take

anything, nor do I have a dermatologist. Should I?' I was aware that we were ignoring the patient, who was still waiting outside the room, but I felt like I needed to get my name added to the dermatologist's clinic list for my own consultation.

We both sat down. He didn't seem at all fazed by the waiting patient. Instead, he was excited, as though I was some medical marvel. He reassured me that I didn't need to be treated by a specialist, but most people with skin like mine insisted on being seen, at least for a few appointments, to understand it better, and he suggested that I take daily antihistamines to dampen down my hyperactive skin reactions. I instantly and politely told him that I'd prefer not to do so.

He pondered on this for a few moments, and then concluded that if I had managed this far without medication, I would likely be OK. He took the end of his own pen and made a mark on the back of my other hand. At the end of our conversation, he examined the neat line of swelling that he had made with a satisfied smile.

'Just marvellous!' he concluded. I had never before felt so proud of my own anatomy.

That was how I received my diagnosis of dermatographic urticaria, or dermatographia. Some people prefer the less clinical term of 'skin writing'.

Due to the skin condition I now knew to be dermatographia, along with some facial acne that I'd suffered with since my late teens, dermatology was the only placement in which I felt I had some personal experience and could relate a little to the patients. There were things that I already knew about the skin, different conditions and treatments, so for once, I wasn't starting off at ground zero.

For my dermatology placement at Red Hospital, my supervising consultant that was assigned to me, wasn't able to supervise me every single day due to unexpected commitments, so kindly arranged for me to be supervised by the registrar on the dermatology team. I didn't mind at all. At this stage in my placement rotations, I was more than used to working with whoever was happy to have me, with or without a prior introduction.

The registrar supervising me became the person I spent most of my placement with, which I enjoyed. Towards the end, it felt more like working each day with a friend as opposed to a supervisor who would be assessing me and signing me off as competent when the clinical placement finished. If she felt that was true, which I really hoped she did.

The registrar appeared much younger than I had expected, compared to the registrars I had spent time with on my previous placements. She spoke with a heavy American accent, which I liked as it reminded me of my American Godparents in Colorado, who I didn't get to see as often as I would have liked to. She had been working in the dermatology department for some time and was extremely experienced and knowledgeable in all things skin, yet seemed relaxed and laid back in her approach and attitude. Despite me being provided with a timetable for the clinics that I would attend and shadow each day whilst I was in the department, she made sure that I was happy with how my time was divided up. She begged me to ask questions if I ever had any, stressing that there was no such thing as a silly question. I loved her energy.

She was a similar height to me, and quite slim in build. As a result, I was surprised when she told me that she was a competitive weightlifter, apologising in advance for any strong-smelling lunches, often consisting of eggs, fish or both, as she tried to maximise her protein intake.

Despite being great at her job, she was the kind of doctor who didn't want her role to define who she was as a person, and actively pursued many other passions and hobbies outside of the dermatology ward. She was actually the first experienced doctor I worked with who reminded me that being a clinician is great, but we are also allowed to have an entire existence outside of the clinical walls. And whilst this had always been true and even told to us in our lectures, my own existence had become so encompassed in textbooks, the *British National Formulary* *(BNF)*, medical revision and clinical placements, I had forgotten that once qualified, I was going to be as free as a bird, at least outside of my working hours.

When the registrar asked me what my own hobbies were, surprisingly, I had forgotten what I used to do before this intensive course took over my life. Reading, writing, travelling, photography and, more recently, running. These were things I had enjoyed, but hadn't done for such a long time.

One of the things that caught my attention was that my supervisor had the most perfect blemish-free and almost glowing skin. At this stage, I was still trying to keep my acne under control, and failing somewhat miserably. Most people I knew developed acne during puberty and into their mid-teens, but at that time, my skin remained perfect. It was in my late teens and early 20s that my skin started to misbehave and the acne arrived.

Along with over-the-counter acne creams, lotions and potions, I had tried dietary changes, drinking more of this, eating less of that, but my skin was as stubborn as I was. Everyone wants to have great skin. Men want to have complexions that are rugged and clear. Women want to be asked 'Are you wearing foundation?' and try not to burst with pride as they casually answer, 'Nope, this is my natural face.' I, on the other hand, just wanted not to have large, painful spots taking up permanent residence on my face.

My own acne had made me subconsciously drawn to other people's skin as I absentmindedly stared in jealous admiration at their spot-free faces and wondered if they perhaps knew something that I didn't. I asked the registrar what products she used on her face and she told me that she took Roaccutane. I knew a little about this hardcore acne drug from university lectures and my own learning, but up to now, I'd always ended up persuading myself against it.

Roaccutane is the brand name of the isotretinoin drug used to treat severe acne that hasn't responded to other treatments. It works by reducing the oil produced in the glands, which in turn reduces the blockage of pores and consequently eliminates spots. The drug is effective, but very strong, and can only be prescribed by specialist dermatologists.

The Roaccutane clinic would be one of the first places that I shadowed the registrar and I was excited to see just how effective this magical drug really was. Instead of reading reviews on Google and watching videos of strangers' thoughts on YouTube, I would be able to get a front-row seat of the results.

Whilst they're taking the drug, it is compulsory for patients to have regular blood tests to keep an eye on things like cholesterol, the liver and kidneys. Monitoring of mental health is also important, as a potential side effect of this drug is mood deterioration. And under no circumstances is a female patient taking this medication to get pregnant. A child conceived by a mother taking Roaccutane would likely be born with severe birth defects affecting their major organs. An infant fathered by someone taking the drug wouldn't have any health problems at all. This meant that a woman had to be on at least one method of contraception before the drug was even prescribed.

The Roaccutane clinic was held in one of the dermatology rooms which looked a lot like a smaller version of a GP's consulting room. It was white and clean with a desk and computer for the doctor to use and a couple of seats in front of this for the patient, a small examination couch and sink on the far wall. Before the clinic began, I took one of the chairs to my usual spot of imagined invisibility in the corner of the room.

Each patient had a red A4 cardboard folder with their name on it, containing sheets of paper documenting previous dermatology consultations, along with their original referral letter from their GP. These folders made me feel useful and gave me something to do as I hurried to collect each one from the shelf where they were kept outside the consultation room and give it to the registrar. She would then read it and familiarise herself with each patient's case before calling them into the room.

Most of the patients in the Roaccutane clinic were females. Statistically, females are more likely to suffer with acne requiring a specialist's input than males, due to their hormones. This isn't to say that males do not suffer from acne, as they definitely do. In fact, some of the more severe cases of acne that I witnessed in the Roaccutane clinics afflicted men, but mostly, it was women we saw.

I asked the registrar why she thought this was. She replied that it wasn't clear, but it might be to do with the fact that generally, males would delay going to their GP to ask for help with their skin for longer than females. I thought back to my GP placement and generally, how few patients had been young men compared to young women.

And of those young men, very few came for treatment of acne compared to their female counterparts.

The consultations between the registrar and her male and female patients in the Roaccutane clinic were more or less identical, involving checking recent blood test results, asking about mental health and side effects, how the patient was getting on with the medication and if they felt that it was helping them. The main difference was the females would do a compulsory pregnancy test before their prescription was written. The patient would provide a urine sample in a cup in the toilet, then bring it back to the consultation room where it would be tested on the spot.

Often, I could feel the palpable tension from the patient as she waited to be told if her pregnancy test was negative. Which it should always have been, due to the contraception she'd strictly agreed to take. On one occasion, though, while I was shadowing the registrar in the Roaccutane clinic, a pregnancy test result came back positive. My registrar repeated the test again and again, just in case the batch she was using was faulty, yet each time, the result confirmed, with a faint second pink line, the patient's pregnancy.

Whilst trying to remain calm, the registrar asked the patient about the contraception she was using. Confusingly calm herself, the patient informed us that she had had her coil removed at the sexual health clinic as she felt it was giving her mood swings, and had forgotten to insist her partner wear a condom.

The situation was bad. The patient was asked to wait outside the room whilst the registrar made a call to one of her colleagues. Even though the registrar knew the protocol, this had not happened to her in a long time and she needed to run her plan by her colleague to make sure she was doing the right thing for the patient and recently discovered foetus.

As it turned out, the patient did not want to go through with the pregnancy. However, the usually relaxed registrar seemed troubled by the whole situation. After the patient had left, having discussed her options regarding the unwanted pregnancy and taken leaflets of advice and directions to the sexual health clinic nearby, I asked the registrar why she felt as she did. She explained that if the patient had wanted to go through with the pregnancy, it would have been a very difficult situation, likely ending in termination anyway due to the strength of the dose of Roaccutane that the patient was currently taking daily. We discussed the fact that the patient had, in a sense, 'gone rogue'. Despite having agreed to remain on contraception during her treatment, she had stopped taking it without discussing it with either the registrar or her GP. This was a situation that the registrar could have neither predicted nor prevented.

After a debrief and a deep breath, we called in our next patient and the registrar apologised for keeping him waiting. A male in his early 30s, he was highly unlikely to be pregnant, which was a relief as we couldn't take any more drama for the rest of the clinic.

Skin cancer seemed to be the main health concern in the specialty as it was the focus and feature of most of the posters decorating the walls in the dermatology department. There are two different types of non-melanoma skin cancer, basal cell carcinoma, appearing as a small pearly lump, and squamous cell carcinoma, which resembles more of a raised pink lump, often with crusting on the surface.

Both of these lesions, when identified, require a referral to dermatology. Therefore, these were the types of lesions I saw with the dermatologist in the skin cancer clinic. The referrals came from general practice with the patient raising their concern with their GP, and the GP referring them to dermatology for a closer examination and specialist diagnosis.

The consultation room for this was a little larger than that of the acne clinic, as more space was required to examine the patient's body with ease. Some of the lesions of concern were in difficult-to-see places, requiring the patient to be in various positions and states of undress. With some patients, the GP had come to an almost certain conclusion they had skin cancer that needed to be verified via a process called a biopsy before treatment was initiated. Others had skin lesions and marks that even I, as a student, could tell weren't skin cancer, but they had been referred as it is better to get a specialist opinion, just to be safe. And then there was the sweet elderly lady who walked into the consultation room after being called by the registrar with a large and obvious squamous cell carcinoma sitting on the side of her nose like an unsightly oversized stud.

Even though the patient's notes contained the original referral letter, detailing the reason for her clinic attendance, it was good practice to take a brief history, just to hear the situation in her own words. She explained that she had had this 'beauty spot' on her nose for the past few months and it was slowly getting bigger. She took it as a symptom of getting older and didn't worry too much about it. However, her daughter had visited and told her that she didn't like the look of it and she should show it to her GP. Her GP didn't like the look of it either, and subsequently referred her to the clinic, urgently.

Despite the lesion being huge, the registrar examined it closely under the dermatoscope. She then confirmed the suspicion we both had that the lesion was most likely to be a squamous cell carcinoma, but that would need to be confirmed by taking a small sample and sending it to the lab to be examined in a biopsy.

This was explained to the patient. 'Oh no, dears, I don't want my beauty spot removed,' she replied in alarm. 'It's part of me now. I only came so that I could say to my daughter I took her advice and attended. But honestly, I'd prefer to keep my little beauty spot, if it's all the same to you.'

The registrar and I exchanged surprised glances, without saying a word. The patient had been counselled by her GP about the high likelihood of this being a type of skin cancer, and looking at it, I realised it met all of the specific criteria. This was reiterated by the registrar, who said that there was a small chance it would worsen and spread. The patient appeared to understand this, and as she had full mental capacity, she was free to make her own decisions about what she felt was best for her health, treatment and care. The registrar and I were merely guides ensuring that she had all the information she needed to make an informed decision.

In the end, after briefly summarising her concerns to the patient, the registrar decided that we had reached as far as we could go in this consultation. The patient was given some information leaflets and advised to attend a follow-up appointment to reassess the lesion and see if she had changed her mind about having it removed. She politely but firmly told us that she would take the appointment if we insisted, but she wouldn't be changing her mind. She then thanked us for our time and gave us each a fruit flavoured boiled sweet, accepted the leaflets and a written summary of the consultation, and left.

Minor procedures, which reminded me of the children's game Operation, were commonplace in dermatology. A small incision, an eye for precision and a steady hand were all essential for the successful removal of a lump, bump or anything else growing underneath or on top of the skin that shouldn't be there.

Within dermatology, there was a fine line between

procedures that were allowed to be carried out as part of medical treatments on the NHS, and those that were purely cosmetic and needed to be paid for and carried out by a private healthcare clinic. A tiny lump on the leg that had been present for a decade and not caused any symptoms during that time, once it was cleared of being anything of concern, would likely not be eligible to be removed on the NHS. A lump causing pain or discomfort, or that was large or awkward enough to catch on things causing bleeding and wounds, would be looked into and was more likely to be treated or removed on the NHS.

The difficulty, however, was the subjectivity of it all. Some patients chose to tolerate things that definitely could be treated and fixed on the NHS, others struggled to manage things that most people would not have even noticed. Neither type of patient was right or wrong, everybody's just different. It was important to advise patients that even if they hadn't decided whether they wanted treatment or removal, they should get all lumps and bumps reviewed by their GP, to be on the safe side.

Minor dermatological procedures didn't need the large operating theatres I had grown so accustomed to, with the big overhead lights and a whole team of staff standing around the patient's bed. Instead, they could take place in one of the dermatology clinic rooms. These had an adjustable table for the patient to lie on, but were far more simple. However, there were lots of interesting cupboards and drawers around the rooms, filled with all the types of equipment and dressings essential to the specialty. I enjoyed looking through the cupboards when there was no patient present, trying to work out what each strangely shaped object was used for.

One of the patients booked into the minor procedure clinic was coming in for the removal of a cyst on his upper back. The cyst had repeatedly become infected and treated with antibiotics over time. Although the size of a golf ball, it was not currently infected, but it was still causing the patient so much discomfort, he had even had to alter the position in which he slept at night.

I had seen a cyst removed before, but wasn't completely confident in my ability to stomach what I was about to witness, as this one was so large. The patient lay down on his front on the tissue-covered couch with his shirt off and his head facing towards his left shoulder, in the direction of where I was standing. The registrar had readied all of her equipment on a shiny wheeled metal trolley at her side. The patient's back was covered with a large white sheet, into which she had made a small hole that she carefully placed over the cyst, exposing it to us.

Whilst local anaesthetic was injected under his skin in different areas around the cyst, the patient began to tell me about his morning in response to me asking if he was alright. I had been worried that the large needle in his back might be too much for him to bear. He was a chatty man, but I was unsure whether this was just his personality, or a result of nerves about having the skin of his back cut open whilst he was wide awake. Either way, I was happy to engage him in conversation and learn about the mischief of his dog, who had chewed the toes of his favourite formal leather shoes earlier in the day.

The registrar, interrupting the story, informed him that she would be touching different areas on his back and he should let her know if he felt anything. As she applied pressure with the needle, she did it heavily enough that he would be able to feel the sharp stimulus if the anaesthetic wasn't working, but lightly enough to ensure she didn't puncture the skin unnecessarily. Once the patient had confirmed that he was unable to feel anything at all, the procedure began.

With the scalpel, the registrar gently made short strokes along the centre of the bulging cyst, almost as if she was sketching with a pencil. The strokes were skilful, always in the exact same place, meaning every one cut a little deeper into the skin. I had expected lots of blood, but surprisingly, there wasn't much at all, and the blood that did form was easily dabbed away with the piece of sterile gauze the registrar had placed next to the opened skin.

Once the layer of skin had been cut down to where the cyst began, the registrar asked if I could see it. I didn't know what I was looking at; it just seemed to be an open wound in the middle of the back.

'How about now?' she asked with a cheeky grin, as her hands gently applied pressure to each side of the cyst. What followed was a volcano-like eruption of sebaceous tissue, which I can only describe as looking like perfectly smooth mashed potato. I was as horrified as I was fascinated, but tried to keep the expression on my face positive as the patient lying on his front seemed to be watching me closely for any indication of trouble.

'Yes, I definitely see it now,' I said through a large fake smile.

The registrar used another piece of sterile gauze to half wipe, half grab the soft white contents of the cyst, which was now sitting obediently on the top of the skin. Once this was removed, she applied more pressure and the process repeated until all that was left oozing out was blood. The area of skin on the patient's back looked red from all the pressing and squeezing, but was noticeably flatter without the large lump.

The registrar asked me if I wanted to suture and close the wound, after getting consent from the patient. He said he didn't mind and was actually enjoying lying down, as his puppy had kept him awake during the night. I decided that as much as I was good at suturing, having picked up the technique quickly when it was taught in class on pieces of pig skin, today I would just focus on observing.

The patient was cleaned and stitched up and a dressing was applied. He was then done and free to go, after being given some information on wound management, how to look after the area and when to have the stitches removed at his GP practice. He thanked us and left, leaving us to dispose of his cyst contents, and clean and sterilise the instruments and room. The registrar was so casual and jovial about it all, I wondered if she had always been this way or if her tolerance to unsightly things on the human body had built up over time.

When I was growing up, one of my younger brothers had eczema. Usually, this would be well controlled, but sometimes it would become quite bad, with my parents having to apply different creams, emollients and topical steroids throughout the day, and sometimes the night.

When we were young, he used to ask me to help him scratch his itchy skin, and I was happy to in return for different favours such as picking the Disney video we would watch next. We had to scratch in secret as our parents were always telling him that he mustn't, because his skin was starting to bleed in places. I focused my charity scratches particularly on his back, which he struggled to reach. It was the least a big sister could do.

As I've become older, I've started to understand that with eczema and dermatitis – the itchiness of the skin that makes you want to scratch – the process of scratching actually makes it more itchy. This is called the itch-scratch cycle and is something, unbeknownst to me at the time, I unfortunately helped keep my brother trapped in.

Because of my brother's eczema, I grew up knowing what this condition looks like on darker skin. My mixed-race cousin also suffered badly, and it was interesting to compare how different the eczema looked on them due to the differences in their complexions. It was similar with the acne that I had suffered. The scars it occasionally left would look like little dark marks dotted across my face. On a lighter skin complexion, those acne scars would likely be red, pink, or even white.

During my dermatology placement and my own medical revision, I became aware that different skin complaints and diseases only tended to be shown in pictures in the textbooks on Caucasian skin tones. I worried that students like myself might not learn how different dermatological conditions could look on darker complexions, potentially leading to misdiagnoses or delays in prescribing important treatments. Even common childhood illnesses like chicken pox look very different on a white child, an Asian child and black child. And whilst the difference in the complexions that make up the multicultural society in the UK is something to be celebrated, I worried about the potential for unintentional disadvantages towards darker skinned people.

My supervising registrar and the other dermatologists I shadowed within the department were extremely knowledgeable and experienced at identifying skin conditions and diseases on all skin tones, likely because of the diversity in the population of Tooting Broadway. They even taught me valuable differences to look out for. New books and resources like *Mind The Gap*, a free online handbook published by Malone Mukwende, a St George's medical alumnus, and colleagues in 2020, are a step in the right direction in helping to educate clinicians on conditions and diseases in all skin tones, ensuring safe and effective treatment for patients of all ethnicities.

CHAPTER 10

HEADQUARTERS

Our first patient of the day in the ear, nose and throat (ENT) department was a four-year-old girl who had decided, just for fun, to stick a bead into her right ear canal.

The patient entered the room hand in hand with her dad, and the ENT physician associate Vivienne introduced herself and me. After a brief scan of the room, taking in the surroundings, the equipment and a gloved and aproned Vivienne, the patient decided that she would rather be anywhere other than here. Letting go of her dad's hand, she walked briskly out of the still-open door, glancing over her shoulder to see if he would obediently follow. Instead, he gently took her by the shoulders and led her back into the clinical room, closing the door behind them and apologising to us both.

Vivienne continued to smile enthusiastically at the little girl as the patient's father lifted her on to the bed, ignoring his daughter's protests. After some heartfelt promises and bribery from her father, the patient agreed to let us look into her ear and admire her earlier handiwork. She denied any pain, but it was hard to tell if she was telling the truth or just trying to get away from us as fast as possible.

Vivienne slowly and gently inserted the handheld otoscope into the ear, using the camera attachment to display the image clearly on the large screen above the patient's head. A single pink bead, sitting comfortably in the child's small ear canal, came into view. The bead was deep inside, shiny and perfectly round, each of these features increasing its difficulty of removal.

The patient, clearly unsure which emotion to present to us, was flicking her eyes rapidly between myself, Vivienne and her father.

'No tears, please,' he begged his little girl, not backing down. 'I told you that the beads mustn't go in your mouth or your ears, yet you insisted, and this is the consequence.'

'I want to go home now. Please, I'm sorry,' the patient responded.

'I know that you're sorry, pumpkin, but the bead still has to be removed. It can't stay there forever.'

'Why not? Mum has earrings, this can be mine.' This made me laugh, which unfortunately made the little girl cry. I wanted to explain that I wasn't mocking her, but rather laughing at her quick wit. However, I knew at this point that the game was over.

Vivienne, who was relying on the patient to keep her

head perfectly still, was struggling. The child had decided that she wanted Vivienne to stop, so was moving her head from left to right, leaving Vivienne with no option but to remove the otoscope from the ear entirely so as not to cause damage. Vivienne tried another approach, gentle persuasion, explaining that the little bead had to come out so that it wouldn't make her ear poorly. But the more Vivienne talked, the more the patient wailed. When her dad tried to comfort her, she wailed even louder. It might have been three adults in a battle of wills with one small human being, but it seemed that we had lost.

Dad, raising his voice above his daughter's cries, asked Vivienne what would happen next. Vivienne explained that the only viable next step would be to have the bead removed with the patient under general anaesthetic. Despite its guarantee of success, it was an outcome that Vivienne had clearly been hoping to avoid. Any procedure using general anaesthesia takes time, costs money and isn't without its risks, and this patient was still so very young.

Once Vivienne had explained all this to the patient's dad, he asked if he could make a quick call to his wife. After outlining the situation to her, he passed the phone to his still sobbing daughter so she could talk to her mummy. We then listened in to one side of the subsequent conversation.

'But I don't want to... I want to go home... Noooooo!' It was clear that the patient was having none of it and would need to be booked on to the list for general anaesthetic and foreign body removal. It was at that point I realised I am one of those peculiar people who finds the prospect of watching the removal of things from ears somewhat satisfying, and I wondered if I would still be on this ENT placement when the little patient received her appointment.

Otology is the branch of medicine focusing on the ear. Rhinology focuses on the nose, and sinuses and laryngology on the upper airway structures in the throat. Most doctors within ENT are otolaryngologists, working in all three specialties combined.

These three specialties have always been grouped together like triplets because of the close proximity of the ear, nose and throat to each other, leading to some occasional crossover symptoms. Whilst the ear, nose or throat may be seen as lesser structures, they are extremely important for the entire body. Ears are responsible for hearing, as everyone knows, but also play a key role in balance and coordination, helping us walk straight without bumping into things or other people. The nose is responsible for smell, but also helps us to taste and breathe. And without a throat, we wouldn't be able to taste or breathe, or talk and swallow.

My ENT clinical supervisor was a warm, bubbly middle-aged man, always wearing a big toothy smile as if there was nowhere else he would rather be than on the hospital wards. With the extensive experience he had, this may have been true. Not only was he an ENT consultant, he was also a head and neck plastic surgeon, and a consultant in the nearby eye hospital. He had worked all over the world and seemed to have been born to do his job.

I love working with people who are paid to do what appears to be a personal hobby rather than just a job. They inspire me. Whilst he was explaining that I would be spending time with different colleagues of his, as well as with him, he encouraged me to give feedback on anything that I would like to do more or less of while I was in the department.

At the time, ENT at Green Hospital was a specialty that already had fully qualified physician associates working within it, meaning that they had done all the groundwork in explaining the role to other staff members and patients, so I didn't have to. It also meant that I was able to see exactly where a physician associate would fit into the department and what we could be working on day to day, just like in AMU.

Vivienne was one of the first clinicians I was timetabled to shadow in ENT. She was well known to us physician associate students, as she had been involved in our lectures and practical sessions on the course. Young but authoritative, she appeared to be well-liked and respected by her colleagues on the ward.

Any physician associates actively working in the profession were held up almost as mini-celebrities by us students. It felt special to see and speak to people doing a job that no-one else really knew much about at the time, whilst we were all taking the risk to train to become one of them anyway. It was exciting and validating, but also a bit intimidating, knowing that after graduating, we would work alongside these physician associates and be expected to measure up to the same high standards they had set.

If I hadn't known Vivienne from the course, I would have assumed that she was one of the registrars within the department. She knew so much and was extremely confident in herself and her ability, whilst remaining humble and approachable. The gap between where she was in her career and where I was as a student seemed impossible to bridge. I had to keep reminding myself that she had been working full time for a few years and one day, I too would be as confident and, more importantly, competent.

Despite not being my supervisor, Vivienne was always checking in and making sure that I was doing OK and experiencing all the things that I wanted and needed to during my time on ENT. I vowed that when I qualified, I would be sure to take extra care of physician associate students that I might work with, just as Vivienne had looked after me.

The ENT clinical room in which I had my first shadowing session was similar to all the others in all the specialties I had seen so far. It was a standard size with a bed in the centre, but suspended above where the patient's head would lie was a large screen. Vivienne explained that it helped her see inside the patient's ear, and I would be able to watch and see what she was doing as she slowly and carefully inserted a long, narrow device with a tiny camera on the end.

I was thrilled at this as I had been expecting only to hear a verbal report of what she was seeing after each examination. Instead, I would be able to watch the live footage of the examination as it happened.

If a patient is referred to the ENT department for earwax removal, it generally means that it is a difficult case, as wax is usually removed quickly and easily in general practice by water irrigation. Sometimes, though, a patient's ear drum, canal or medical history means that water irrigation should be avoided and microsuction is more appropriate.

Microsuctioning is exactly as it sounds. A small, thin tube-like device is inserted into the ear canal and gently sucks up and removes wax, debris, discharge and sometimes foreign bodies like a little pink bead. It makes a noise similar to a vacuum cleaner and I wondered how the patient would feel, having this directly inside their ear during the wax removal.

One of the patients I saw with Vivienne was an elderly gentleman. He loved to swim for fitness and enjoyment, but recent ear infections had forced him to stop. His left ear had become painful and was discharging gunky fluid, but his symptoms weren't responding to or improving with the antibiotic tablets and drops given to him by his GP. Therefore, he was sent to ENT for further examination and advice.

The patient was very friendly. Despite being in his 80s, he looked much younger, and I told him so. He returned the favour by mentioning that I looked too young to be a medical student (or equivalent). I was aware of this and didn't love to be reminded, but tried to take it as the compliment he'd intended.

Vivienne changed the tip of the otoscope whilst explaining that she wanted to remove some of the debris. She then introduced the microsuction device inside the ear, sucking out fungal debris, which revealed why the antibiotic treatment hadn't been working as the patient didn't have a bacterial ear infection at all. Bacterial infections tend to cause thick discharge inside the ears, often yellow and green coloured. But when the fungal debris was removed from the patient's ears by the microsuction device, it reminded me of dusty cobwebs from the corners of the ceiling. The fungal spores made my skin crawl a little. They were white with black spots, looking like small balls of Dalmatian-like cotton wool sitting inside the ear canal.

When all the fluffy debris had been sucked up and removed from the patient's ear canal, Vivienne explained that she still wanted him to use antifungal eardrops for a few more days. After arranging the prescription, she handed it to the patient. Relieved to be turning a corner and hoping to get back in his beloved swimming pool in the near future, he thanked us both, tipping his hat to us in turn, then went on his way.

. . .

When people attended the ENT department for a problem with their nose, it was commonly the sinuses within the face causing the problem. They could either be blocked, infected or both. Occasionally, though, people would have problems with the nose itself, its alignment causing them trouble with breathing. Any issues to do with the skin on the outside of the nose tended to be treated by the dermatologist. The ENT consultants were only really interested in the inside of the nose.

During my GP placement, nasal examinations merely consisted of me shining a medical torch up inside the nose, trying to see as far as I could. Which, incidentally, wasn't that far. The ENT department, however, had lots of fascinating specialist equipment, allowing for a much greater range of vision and clarity in places that were difficult to access.

A nasendoscopy is one procedure that particularly impressed me. It involves a handheld device with a round eyepiece on one end. On the other end of the fist-sized device is a long, flexible piece of what looks like narrow black tubing, which can be inserted not merely into the nostrils, but all the way down to the back of the throat. When the clinician looks down the eyepiece, they are able to have a perfect view and carry out a thorough examination, easily identifying any abnormalities present.

One of the first ENT surgical procedures I observed was for a patient who had been suffering with chronic sinusitis. I'd never had sinusitis myself, but remembered from my GP placement how unwell it could make people.

The sinuses are empty spaces behind the cheekbones and in the forehead, allowing a small amount of mucus to form, keeping the area moisturised. The mucus present also protects the sinuses from dirt, dust and microorganisms. On occasions, though, an infection can develop inside these spaces, causing swelling, increased mucus and pain.

If the patient is very unfortunate, they will find themselves stuck in a vicious cycle of infection, inflammation, swelling, narrowing, blocking, and then more infection. Symptoms can include severe headaches, blocked nose, nasal discharge, but mostly awful pain across the face and teeth, which can be so debilitating that the patient is unable to continue with their normal day-to-day activities. If the problem is ongoing and the usual treatment of steam, steroid nasal spray and oral antibiotics doesn't help, then surgical intervention can sometimes be required.

My supervisor showed me a CT scan of the head of the patient we were about to operate on. With other medical imaging I had seen, it tended to be quite obvious what body part I was looking at. X-ray images in particular were fairly easy to determine, because the outline of the body remained present, even if just faintly. CT scans, on the other hand, were much more difficult to understand and interpret.

On X-ray images, the bones are shown as white against the black background. With CT scans, the bones are still white, but air is seen as black, and soft tissue and fluids are grey, meaning that there is a lot more to interpret in the image. The CT scan of the head that my consultant was showing me looked quite frightening, with hollowed-out facial spaces like a skull and bulging grey eyes. Incidentally, neither of these appearances was abnormal; the consultant just wanted to show me the pockets of fluid in the patient's sinuses, something I hadn't yet seen and wouldn't have noticed otherwise.

The consultant was extremely excited as he explained that during the procedure, his job was to remove all of the mucus trapped in the sinuses, along with swollen tissue and any other obstructions, allowing the sinuses to clear and drain. This was to be done via a process called an antral lavage, or sinus washout. It was a pretty simple procedure in essence, with more of a focus on symptom control than a long-term solution.

With the patient fast asleep on the table, a thin telescopic instrument was inserted into the nostrils with a tiny camera projecting the image on to a nearby screen. Whilst the removal of the mucus was simple and straightforward, during the procedure, the consultant found a small piece of bone, only millimetres in size, that he believed to be a contributing factor as to why the patient kept getting infections. The consultant wanted to remove it.

Due to my aversion to broken bones, I tried to rationalise and tell myself the handheld instruments that resembled a chisel and hammer were only removing a small piece. What I hadn't expected was to be able to hear so loudly and clearly the sound of that small piece of bone being chiselled away. The metal instrument against the bone produced a surprisingly loud tapping noise and I couldn't help worrying that we were going to wake the patient up.

After just moments of tapping and chiselling, the offending piece of bone was dropped with a clink into the shiny silver kidney dish nearby. I found it remarkable how strong bone is and how a piece only a little bigger than a grain of rice had caused the patient so many problems and taken so much effort to remove.

After the procedure, the patient had small dissolvable stitches placed into the wounds and a cotton tampon-like dressing was gently inserted into each nostril, where it was to remain until the bleeding had stopped. The surgery had been a success and the patient was wheeled round to recovery, where he would slowly start to wake up and receive feedback on the positive outcome of his procedure.

A couple of days later, I was asked to accompany a consultant to A&E to review an ENT patient. When we arrived, we found, sitting in one of the cubicles, the same patient I'd seen in surgery. He had his head bent backwards, staring at the ceiling, one hand pinching the bridge of his nose and the other holding a blood-soaked towel. He looked like he had been brutally attacked with the blood smeared on his cheeks, staining his clothing and his hands.

It turned out the patient, thinking that he had inhaled a fly, blew his nose violently, dislodging one of his stitches and causing a heavy nosebleed that had not yet stopped. I must have looked alarmed as the consultant reassured me that bleeding was always quite significant after a procedure, though easily resolved.

The patient was wheeled round to the ENT department and his nostrils were examined using the equipment there. The offending blood vessels were cauterised to stop the bleeding, then more tampon-style dressings were inserted into his nostrils. Finally, the patient was given information and advice on how to look after his nose for the next few weeks.

Tonsillitis is another common ENT infection that I had regularly seen on my GP placement. This affects the tonsils, the two lumps of tissue either side of the throat. When infected, these swell and cause the patient pain, particularly with swallowing.

The infection is often viral, though it can also be bacterial, which causes the tonsils to be covered in thick bad-smelling white pus. Whether the infection is bacterial or viral, it causes significant pain and discomfort for the patient, but whilst viral tonsillitis usually self-resolves in a few days with rest and pain relief, bacterial tonsillitis often requires antibiotics, along with fluids and pain relief.

On rare occasions, what starts out as a simple bacterial tonsillitis ends up having unexpected and life-threatening consequences. If the bacteria causes an abscess to develop on one of the tonsils, this results in a large collection of pus forming between the tonsil and the lining of the throat. This is called a quinsy. The collection of pus then starts to protrude inwards, narrowing the airway inside the throat, limiting the patient's ability to breathe.

The tonsillitis that I had seen on my GP placement was always the straightforward bacterial or viral version, but in our lectures, we were taught the importance of distinguishing between bad tonsillitis and quinsy. And if we ever suspected a quinsy, we were to send the patient straight to A&E without delay as it was a medical emergency.

In ENT, the consultant that I was shadowing one day was bleeped to come to A&E to examine a patient, a female in her late 20s with a suspected quinsy. As we entered her curtained-off bed space, I could tell she wanted to greet us with a smile and hello, but just didn't have it in her. She looked pale and tired, and her facial expression was of someone in a lot of pain. When she went to speak, her voice was high pitched and nasally, making her sound like Daffy Duck. Instead of swallowing her saliva, which had become agonising, the patient had resorted to spitting into a disposable cardboard kidney dish that she was clutching close to her chest.

She was with her mother who gave us the history. The consultant then purposely asked the patient a few closed questions so that she could answer them by either nodding or shaking her head. She had a high fever and pulse rate, was pale and sweaty and had an airway that was becoming increasingly compromised as time went by.

The patient urgently needed surgery for a quinsy.

Whilst she was added on to the emergency list and

prepped for surgery, I was able to change into scrubs and wait for her with the rest of the team in the ENT surgical department. The abscess was large on her right tonsil, almost completely touching her left tonsil. The aim of the procedure was to make an incision in the tonsillar abscess, and then drain away the pus inside as quickly and carefully as possible. This would reduce the protrusion, which would then no longer compromise the patient's airway.

The patient remained awake during the procedure, but was sedated to help her relax and was given local anaesthetic to numb the affected area. She was lying on her back on the trolley in the operating theatre, with her mouth open as wide as the quinsy would allow, and I could now fully see the extent of the problem. Her throat looked like she had a shiny red golf ball sitting on her right tonsil, drastically reducing the space through which she could breathe. Though the mass looked solid, the consultant was certain that it was in fact filled with thick fluid pus and all that was required was for the pus to be removed.

With a wooden depressor pushing firmly down on the patient's tongue, the consultant inserted a large hand-held syringe with a long, wide silver needle attached to the end into her mouth. He then asked me if I was ready, but without waiting for my response, he slowly introduced the needle into the abscess. As more and more of the needle sank into the abscess, I wasn't sure what to expect. Perhaps an explosion of pus similar to popping a ripe facial pimple. But in this instance, nothing happened.

'Now, watch this,' said the consultant, as if reading

my mind and sensing my disappointment. He removed the wooden tongue depressor, freeing up his hand to pull back the plunger of the syringe, leaving the needle deep within the abscess. Without delay, the clear syringe tube inside the patient's open mouth started to fill with thick custard-like discharge, whilst the abscess slowly shrank. It was satisfying to watch and I thought about the relief that the patient would be experiencing, even under sedation.

After all the pus was drained, the syringe was slowly removed from the abscess and the patient's mouth, leaving only a slight area of redness and a small bead of blood in its place. I had expected more brutality, whilst at the same time being impressed by how civilised the procedure had been.

As the patient had such a high fever and the initial abscess had been so large, she was to have additional antibiotics administered through her veins as a precaution. She would spend the night in hospital for rest and recovery, but in the long run, she was going to be fine.

Within the ENT specialties, and the surgical procedures that go with them, it is interesting to notice the difference between them all. Ear procedures tend to be extremely slow and gentle. The ear canal and eardrum are delicate structures requiring lots of care.

Procedures on the throat are also done gently. The throat tissue is soft and bleeds easily, the airways need to be constantly monitored and the teeth must be protected from accidental cracks and breaks during the surgery.

Nasal procedures, on the other hand, whilst still done with the highest level of care and attention, are definitely more rough. This is because the nose is a bony structure, and for a healthy person, its bones are very strong.

The most difficult procedure for me to observe on the ENT placement was a septorhinoplasty, more commonly known as a nose job. Typically, procedures like septorhinoplasty are not carried out on the NHS as they are considered to be cosmetic and for appearance only. In some cases, however, it is the only treatment option.

This was the case for my next patient. He'd suffered a sporting accident resulting in a broken nose a few years ago, but he had decided to let the nose heal by itself without medical intervention. Whilst it did heal, it was left leaning off to one side. The leaning had worsened with time, meaning that the patient was now struggling to breathe through his nostrils as the space had become constricted.

Whilst he found breathing problematic all year round, it became almost unbearable throughout the summer months with the addition of bad hay fever. The patient was also losing his ability to smell and taste, and life was becoming more and more miserable. Oral medication and steroid nasal sprays hadn't helped, so after graduating from university, he decided to get help.

He'd booked an appointment with his GP, who had referred him to the ENT consultants. After trialling more medication without success, the GP had decided surgery was the only way forward. This was what led to me being in the operating theatre, waiting with some trepidation to observe my first nose job taking place.

A wide incision was made across the patient's septum, which is the tissue separating the two nostrils, the area people sometimes have pierced. I then watched wide eyed as my consultant lifted the skin from the nose and peeled it back, fully exposing the cartilage underneath. The consultant used his hands to manipulate the nasal cartilage back into a straight position, and then the skin was gently laid back. Finally, the wound at the septum was stitched up and the procedure was finished. It was quite horrific to witness, although I couldn't help but marvel at modern medicine and the things that could be achieved.

When he was awake again, the patient was advised how long to keep on the cast covering his nose, which would allow it to heal straight, and on general recovery. Under no circumstances was the patient to blow his nose, no matter how many flies he might suspect he'd inhaled.

Working in ENT during my studies has helped me to rationalise with patients since I fully qualified, particularly younger patients who want to have private cosmetic procedures carried out. The nose in particular seems to be a source of lots of patients' unhappiness and dissatisfaction with their facial appearance. Due to the procedures I have been able to witness, especially the ones that didn't quite go to plan, I can discuss with the patient how they would be carried out, along with the potential risks. And whilst the exact explanation will come from the surgeon if they still wish to go ahead, at least I am able to provide them with something to think about in the meantime.

ENT is a unique specialty in that a problem in any or all of the divisions has the potential to dramatically affect a patient's quality and enjoyment of life. ENT issues can prevent a patient from hearing music, dancing, singing, talking, tasting, smelling, participating in sports. Sometimes, the patient's desperation regarding a seemingly trivial ENT issue is a result of the symptoms affecting or preventing them from doing the things they truly love.

Practising medicine isn't always about treating illness and disease. It's also about ensuring that the patient is able to enjoy as many of the things they love as possible, something that we can easily take for granted when we're fit and well.

CHAPTER 11

BLEEP TEST

My liaison psychiatry clinical supervisor was a young consultant with positive energy and a clear passion for his chosen profession. He appeared to be quiet and down to earth, happy to be at work each day. On the first day of my liaison psychiatry placement, he wore metallic silver trainers, which worked well with the rest of his trendy outfit of chinos and a bright, busy shirt. Immediately after our introductions, I complimented his choice of footwear, as I really did like them.

Coming towards the end of my second year of placements, I was looking forward to graduating, finding a job and finally receiving a salary where I would be able to treat myself to whatever I wanted, no longer constrained by the student budget lifestyle. I often found myself looking at other people's clothes, accessories and general possessions for inspiration for my first salary treat. He thanked me and informed me that I too could wear trainers on this placement if I wanted. The team was not strict with the dress code. So long as our clothing was clean and neat, everything was fine.

I was unsure if he had mistaken my compliment for a hint that I too wanted to wear trainers, but after brief consideration the following morning, I decided to stick to my sensible flat black shoes, instead of my maroon high-top Converse, my current favourite go-to footwear. I still looked like a bright-eyed, fresh-faced student, when the image I was going for was the serious, professional physician associate with plenty of experience behind me. I wanted to introduce myself and leave both colleagues and patients shocked that I wasn't already qualified, considering my wisdom, knowledge and professionalism beyond my years. Brightly coloured Converse probably wouldn't help with this.

The liaison psychiatry department was slightly away from the main hospital in its own little building to the side of the car park. The interior didn't have the usual hospital feel to it that I'd become so accustomed to, and seemed more like a corporate office space. There wasn't the clinical smell in the air, there were no shiny white floors and painted walls; in fact, the department even had carpet. The rest of the team all seemed extremely cheerful and relaxed, which made me wonder if the consultant's positive energy had trickled down to them, or if all the happiest clinicians had gravitated to the same hospital department.

Liaison psychiatry is a subspecialty of psychiatry that involves working collaboratively between general medicine and mental health. The role of the liaison psychiatrist is to review and treat patients within the hospital. Occasionally, after being reviewed by the medical team, a patient may be determined to require a psychiatric assessment alongside their medical care, and then the liaison psychiatrist will be contacted. If the patient is found to be acutely mentally unwell and requiring a longer hospital stay, they are then admitted to a psychiatric ward.

My liaison psychiatry placement nearby at the Grey Hospital. Whilst the walk to placement from my home was nice and short, I made up the rest of my step count throughout the day walking to and from the different wards around the hospital whenever my supervisor received a bleep to alert him that psychiatric input was required. The bleep system was used all over the hospitals I had visited and I had seen it in action many times, but much more so during my liaison psychiatry placement.

I remember on my second day of the placement heading out of the liaison psychiatry department with my supervisor, across the carpark to A&E to see a patient who we had been asked to review. A&E consisted of mainly curtained-off bed spaces, though like most hospitals, the department also had side rooms with doors, providing more privacy. The patient was waiting for us in one of the side rooms, sitting in the armchair next to the hospital bed. In her late teens, she had an expressionless look on her face, and was wearing an oversized hoodie that seemed to swallow her entire body whole, sparing only her head. She wore skinny blue jeans and on her feet were maroon high-top converse. I was extremely grateful for my earlier decision to wear my sensible 'almost fully qualified physician associate' black shoes, as at this moment, I wanted her trust, so needed to look like a clinical professional rather than a peer.

My supervisor knocked on the door, introducing me as a physician associate student, asking if we could both come in and whether she was happy for me to be present during the consultation. She slowly looked me up and down, as I waited anxiously to see if I would pass her unspoken test. After a few seconds, though it felt like an eternity, she gave the slightest of nods in my direction. I thanked her genuinely.

My supervisor and I went to grab two plastic chairs and brought them into her side room, placing them at a far enough distance from her that it didn't seem like we were encroaching on her limited personal space within this room, but close enough that it didn't seem like we were worried about catching something nasty and contagious from her. At the last moment, I decided to move my chair to the corner of the room to have more of a spectator's vantage point, hoping to make the seating plan even less intimidating, though she didn't seem to notice my move at all. She simply gazed downwards, studying her feet.

I watched as my supervisor tried to engage her in conversation and determine what events had led up to her presenting to A&E alone on this weekday morning. He continued to ask questions, pausing to give her the opportunity to respond, but no words came from her, no head gestures or eye contact.

The supervisor finally asked if it would be OK to contact someone for her, to which she whispered, 'My mum, please.'

We left the room and the supervising consultant had a look through her paper file again. She had presented to the A&E department a few times, mainly when she felt suicidal, but wanted to keep herself safe. The consultant then called her mother, who responded that she would leave work immediately and come to the hospital. Despite the patient not giving us any information, she had been able to express her desire for her mum, which might have been all we needed to know. With her mum present, she might feel more comfortable to talk so that we could offer help and support. Still, it got me thinking what the next step would have been if she'd continued not to engage or respond to our questions, or if she hadn't wanted us to call anyone on her behalf.

The next day, my supervisor informed me that the patient had been admitted to the ward overnight, and then discharged home with a plan she had seemed happy with. Members of the home treatment team would visit and support her, ensuring that she got the best help.

Liaison psychiatry was a different type of medicine to what I had become used to. Typically, before each new placement began, I would do as much reading around the common conditions, blood tests and scan results within the specialty as possible, ready for any unexpected questions that may be directed at me on my first day.

Mental-health conditions, however, were typically not diagnosed by blood tests and scans. This was a specialty of watching and listening. Often, the patient alone held all of the information the consultant required, as opposed to the blood tests and scans which were generally invaluable in secondary-care medicine diagnoses. Sometimes additional help was needed from family and friends who might also have important details, but mostly it was a process of piecing together information surrounding the patient's day-to-day life that helped lead to their diagnosis.

Blood tests and scans were still used where needed, but in a different capacity. Liaison psychiatry was more about creating a safe space for the patient to feel free to talk and explain what they had been thinking and feeling. Once detailed information had been gathered, it would be used by a trained professional to undertake a full psychiatric evaluation. This might be possible after a single consultation, or many consultations over time might be required before a diagnosis and treatment plan could be reached. But it was a journey that the clinician and the patient would take together.

The reliance on a patient's history as opposed to blood tests and scans to contribute to their mental-health diagnosis could be helpful or unhelpful, depending on the patient in question. I empathised that it must have felt strange and intrusive to be sitting in an unfamiliar room with a mental-health professional you didn't know, sharing all of your personal thoughts and experiences of concern, perhaps for the first time ever. Some patients' symptoms were frightening, embarrassing and generally unsettling, and it must've taken a lot of courage to discuss them one by one. There were other patients, however, who were simply relieved to have the opportunity to discuss things that they had bottled up for a long time, not knowing where to begin or with whom. There were also patients who wanted support, but wouldn't engage, and these were much harder to help.

Capacity is often mentioned in relation to mental health. In definition, it means someone's ability to understand information, make a decision from that information and communicate their decision. A person can lack capacity long term or short term, for different reasons such as physical or mental illness, medication side effects, a brain injury, or the period of time after being unconscious, such as in a coma. Only a medical professional can assess if someone does or does not have capacity, and if they are found to lack capacity, another person is then permitted to make decisions regarding their care on their behalf, whilst still including them as much as possible. This person can be the patient's doctor or other healthcare professional, social worker or carer. They can also be a friend or family member.

Assessing capacity ensures that a patient is getting the best possible outcome for their health and wellbeing, even if at the time, they cannot support themselves optimally. It is important to assume that a patient has capacity unless there is reasonable doubt to suggest that they do not.

In all medical specialties, the purpose of the consultation between a patient and a clinician is to both gather and give information in a two-way discussion. At the end of the consultation, a patient might readily accept the clinician's proposed treatment plan. Sometimes, they might need some time to think about their options, talk with loved ones and do some reading. Sometimes after a consultation, a patient might prefer to avoid treatment altogether, perhaps to see how their condition progresses or improves with time. Other times, they decline treatment for religious, personal, practical or even financial reasons.

As long as a patient has capacity, it is within their right to accept or decline a clinician's proposed treatment plan. With mental-health treatment plans, whilst the importance of patient autonomy remains the same, capacity assesses whether they are well enough to be able to accept or decline their treatment plan, and it has to be taken into consideration whether the patient will become a harm to themselves or others without the proposed treatment.

A patient had been brought into A&E by the police after his recent break up with his girlfriend had caused a decline in his mental health and he had expressed plans to his family to cause her harm. For additional support, his family called the police, who then brought him into A&E for psychological assessment.

When my supervisor and I arrived in A&E, the patient, a man in his 30s, was pacing up and down in his side room, talking to the voices that he was hearing in his head. These voices were telling him to do violent things to his girlfriend, but he was trying to ignore them and distract himself. The patient was worried that eventually, he would give in and do what the voices told him, just to silence them. He seemed sad, frustrated and angry, but mainly very scared.

After an assessment, my supervisor felt that not only did the patient not have capacity, but he also posed an immediate danger to another person. He therefore was not well enough to be discharged from hospital and would be admitted on to the psychiatric ward. The consultant explained this to the patient, who on hearing it immediately seemed relieved. For the time being, he wasn't having to argue with the voices in his head encouraging him to hurt his ex-girlfriend, but instead would be in a facility where he would be unable to cause harm, even if the voices won. He would be able to receive the right treatment and focus on mending his broken heart.

Sometimes in liaison psychiatry, it was difficult for me to know my place ethically. This wasn't due to my supervisor's neglect, but more my own emotional guilt. As a student shadowing a consultant, especially in more complex cases, I was merely a fly on the wall, an uninvolved spectator. The consultant would always introduce himself to a patient, and then introduce me, asking if they were OK for me to be present. They always said yes, but even with permission, I felt like I was stealing a front-row seat on another person's misery.

I was often faced with an internal dilemma between wanting to give the patient in distress their privacy, whilst also wanting to take it all in and learn as much from the experience as possible, observing my supervisor's body language, tone and even volume of voice in response to the patient's behaviour. I rationalised that whatever I could learn would help my own patients in the future.

But if I was ever to have a mental-health crisis resulting in me being brought into hospital, would I want a student sitting and watching in the corner? Probably not. So I tried to be as invisible yet as useful as I possibly could, on hand with a tissue box and encouraging smile whenever it was required of me.

Whilst most of my supervisor's bleeps were received from the A&E department, occasionally we were required on wards that I wouldn't have expected, like the surgical ward. Surgery to me was cutting open and rummaging around in abdomens. However, I came to learn that sometimes, the requirement for surgery was a direct result of someone's poor mental health.

The patient we were visiting on the surgical ward was a young man who had a history of depression and had decided that he wanted to take his life, so with a kitchen knife, he'd inflicted a deep neck laceration almost from ear to ear. The surgical team had never seen anything like it and were amazed that his injuries, and his blood loss, had not indeed taken his life. They hadn't even caused any long-lasting damage, to the patient's dismay, having missed the vital blood vessels. The patient had been found quickly at his home and paramedics were on the scene only moments later. Surgery was required to close the large wound, but on the whole, physically, he was OK.

When we arrived at the ward, his parents were waiting in the corridor, as he had refused to see them. He had only allowed his older brother at his bedside, but had not spoken much to him either. Every couple of minutes, the patient's mother would beckon the older brother out to the corridor where she and her husband waited and paced anxiously, relaying messages of love and support to her son, who just continued to stare out of the nearby window. The raw devastation of his parents was palpable.

My supervisor acknowledged the parents with a warm non-verbal greeting and walked on to the ward to see his newest patient, with me following behind closely, wondering yet again whether I should wait in the corridor. How was it that a random physician associate student could walk into the patient's ward and be at his bedside, whilst his own parents were forbidden. I felt guilty.

As we introduced ourselves to the patient, the older brother dismissed himself and went to wait with his parents in the corridor. After checking that the patient would be OK with my presence during this initial consultation, my supervisor asked if he would be up for talking. The patient nodded in response to both questions.

'Would you like to tell me a little about what happened, leading up to the moment in the kitchen, in your own words?' my supervisor said gently. I had expected the patient to be a closed book, but he was surprisingly keen to talk and it seemed like he had a lot to get off his chest. He explained that he had been feeling low for a long time and things had just got worse and worse until he decided that he didn't want to live anymore. The patient was living with his parents, who had noticed that he wasn't himself and had been trying to reach out to him and offer him support. They had invited him on drives, walks and day trips, made his favourite meals, offered to book GP appointments and attend with him, everything that they could think of, but the patient had declined them all.

The previous day, his parents had come home and found the patient in the kitchen, lying unresponsive in a pool of his own blood. He felt as though he had failed them, yet unbeknownst to him, they felt like they had failed him too. The patient explained that he couldn't talk to his parents because he could see the hurt that he had caused them, and it was too much to bear, so he had asked them not to visit.

My supervisor in his role of consultant explained that the patient's parents had been spoken by other members of the team, and they understood he was not well and had acted out of a place of desperation. The consultant asked a few more questions about how the patient was feeling right now and what he wanted. He said that he would like to see his parents, but they weren't here. Although the parents had been told that the patient did not want to see them, what he clearly didn't realise was they'd still come to the hospital to sit outside his ward, where they had remained for hours.

When the consultant told him that they were right outside and asked if he wanted them to come in, the patient replied softly, 'Yes please,' between the sobs that he could manage with his freshly dressed neck wound. I looked at my supervisor for permission, and when he gave a nod, I went to get the patient's parents. This situation wasn't about me at all, yet I still felt honoured to be the one to tell them that their son had at last requested to see them.

When I went into the corridor and gently told them what their son had said, they both burst into tears. Relief, fear, devastation, happiness, I didn't want to speculate, but it was likely a mixture of all the above. As they composed themselves and walked on to the ward, leaning on one another for support, physically and emotionally, I decided this time to hang back and remain in the corridor to give them their privacy.

'Thank you, Doctor,' said the patient's older brother. He was standing right next to me, yet I had forgotten about him entirely.

I was determined not to take any credit that wasn't mine. 'You're welcome, but I didn't do anything, and I'm not a doctor, I'm a physician associate student shadowing the consultant,' I explained.

'What's a physician associate?' he asked, a question that I should have been used to by then, but due to the emotional rollercoaster over the past hour, I got completely flummoxed and lost my words altogether. 'Tell me later.' He laughed, making me laugh too. Then he went on to the ward to join his parents at his brother's bedside.

The consultant and I walked back to the department in silence, only broken when he asked me if I was alright. He and the rest of the team often asked me if I was alright. Initially, I felt self-conscious about this, wondering if I didn't look alright, but I later realised that they asked because they were well aware of the emotional toll that their specialty could take. There could be good days and bad days, wins and losses, battles between patients and their clinicians. Not all patients wanted to live, and whilst the medical team were celebrating saving someone's life, that same person might be mourning the death that they were hoping for.

Liaison psychiatry isn't for the faint hearted, though I haven't yet found a specialty within the NHS that is. All its staff in all departments and roles are warriors and super-heroes, in my opinion.

It's a misconception that people who are mentally unwell only feel sad. Some patients can be so extremely happy and excited that the elation in itself puts the individual at risk of harming themselves or others.

Mania is a psychological state that causes a patient to experience euphoria, intense moods, hyperactivity and delusions, and will typically last over a week. Hypomania is similar, but the symptoms usually last just a few days. The symptoms that a person may experience include extreme happiness, increased confidence and sexual energy, excitability, being easily distracted, racing thoughts and difficulty concentrating. The behaviour changes that they may display involve being more physically active than normal, speaking quickly, being very friendly and personable, sleeping little, spending money excessively, losing social inhibitions and taking safety risks. Mania and hypomania are more consistent with mental-health conditions such as schizoaffective, bipolar or seasonal affective disorder and postpartum psychosis.

One of the patients my supervisor and I went to review was brought in to A&E by his friend. He was in his 30s, casually dressed and seemed to be having the time of his life, smiling and laughing away to himself in the A&E side room. My supervisor introduced himself and asked if he could come inside the room, which was occupied by the patient and his worried looking friend.

'Of course you can, man, your girlfriend too!' the patient replied excitedly. 'My room is your room! Can I get you both something to drink?' and he proceeded to get up, I assume to look for beverages to offer us.

'This isn't my girlfriend,' said my supervisor, calm and unfazed as he again introduced himself, and then me, asking if I might shadow him. The patient agreed, his body language that of pure joy. He wore a big grin, his eyes were wide, and he threw his head back, roaring with laughter when no jokes had been made. He sat on the edge of the bed, tapping his foot on the floor and playing with his fingers. Every so often, he would invite us on an adventure with him 'to explore the land'.

Initially, when the patient presented to A&E with his friend, the doctors thought that he might have ingested illicit drugs. But blood results showed that there was nothing in his system and his friend was able to confirm on the patient's behalf that he suffered from bipolar disorder and was currently on a high. Normally, the patient could be coerced into more safe and appropriate ways to spend his day when in a manic phase, but this time, his friend, who was also his flatmate, had struggled to keep him under control and was concerned for his safety.

The patient had wanted to go exploring the underground train tracks, so his friend was able to trick him under the pretence that they were going to visit Tooting Broadway station. He then convinced the patient that he knew a shortcut, which actually led them straight to St George's A&E department. The patient wasn't upset with his friend, just willed him to 'chill out and live a little'.

The consultation was bizarre. The patient's friend looked both tired and worried, whereas the patient seemed like the most chilled and relaxed person in the world. I almost felt jealous of his euphoria and wondered if it felt as good as it looked.

Not long after our consultation, the patient was admitted into the psychiatric ward. He didn't have capacity to make sensible decisions, nor was he likely to be able to keep himself safe. As it turned out, he was known to the mental-health team as this wasn't his first time in A&E this year.

When we discussed the patient's admission to the psychiatric ward, his friend looked relieved and informed us that he would let the patient's father know. Whilst the patient was on the ward, the plan was to find the right balance of medication to reduce his extremes of moods. Historically, after a high, the patient would then fall into a deep depression, with each mood potentially as destructive as the other.

Before joining the physician associate course, I hadn't appreciated that there are more aspects to health than just the physical side. From spending time on my clinical placements over the past two years, I had become used to seeing people who were physically unwell, and often this was clear to identify. These patients would sometimes be bed bound, or if mobile, they would need assistance to move around. Family or staff members would be at their bedside, helping with tasks like eating, drinking and personal care.

In short, the physically unwell generally look unwell. On the other hand, mental illness doesn't have a particular look.

On an A&E trip to review a patient, my supervisor and I were met on the ward by a middle-aged woman in a smart suit. The designer bag on her lap caught my eye as I mentally added it to my list of treats to buy myself with my first pay cheque. I assumed that this lady had accompanied the patient we were to be reviewing, only to realise that she was in fact our patient.

My stereotype of what the mentally ill should look like both caught me off guard and disappointed me, but I would have to deal with that later. The patient looked pleasant, but also restless, like she had other places to be. My supervisor, picking up on this, started the consultation without delay.

The patient explained that her work colleagues had earlier told her she looked agitated. When she was approached by a concerned colleague, she'd immediately burst into tears.

'The voices just won't stop,' she'd told them. Her colleague immediately decided that she needed medical attention and brought her to A&E. This colleague was currently sitting in the hospital's café, where the patient had begged her to wait instead of being with her on the ward.

The patient went on to explain that the voices were not new and she had been hearing them for as long as she could remember, but she'd always felt in control of them and could silence them on demand. Today, however, the voices were less compliant and were filling her head with noise. My supervisor asked lots of specific questions, writing notes ferociously on a piece of paper.

'I was diagnosed with schizophrenia as a teenager,' the patient said casually, making my supervisor stop his frenzied note taking and look up. 'It was manageable then, but it's recently got so much worse. Nobody knows about it. Nobody can know!'

My supervisor looked surprised to realise that the patient already had a mental-health diagnosis. When she had been asked by the A&E doctors in the presence of her colleague whether she had a history of mental illness, she had said that she did not. Only now, with her colleague off the ward, did she feel that she could be honest.

Once again, I felt remorse for assuming that she couldn't be our mental-health patient because of how professionally she was dressed. As a clinician who worked hard to try to avoid prejudice, stereotypes, and bias, I realised that I still had some work to do.

It was decided that the patient would discuss starting medication and ongoing management plans in a follow-up appointment on the ward the next day, and in the meantime, she should go home and rest. She seemed relieved that she would finally be receiving treatment for a condition that she had been trying so desperately to hide from herself and the world.

Mental health as a specialty reminds me of a detective film. Everything is a clue and everything is important, even if it doesn't seem like it at the time. Something may be said by the patient that seems irrelevant, but later turns out to be the very thing that helps to uncover a diagnosis, trigger or past trauma. Active listening, patience, non-judgement, an open mind and good control of facial expressions and body language are all as essential in this specialty as clinical knowledge.

There was still so much for me to learn.

CHAPTER 12

TEST RUN

Clinical placements were not as I had expected them to be. I knew that they were important for learning and putting our lecture-based knowledge into practice. I knew that they were a perfect opportunity for us to interact with real-life patients and not just each other, giving us improved skills in both communication and doing. What I hadn't expected was for my clinical placement experience to be so impactful.

When my clinical placement rotations finished towards the end of the course, it was a bittersweet reality for me. They had provided the perfect combination of working across each clinical specialty, consulting with patients, performing physical examinations and procedures whilst remaining under the protective umbrella of being 'just the student'. As such, our responsibilities were minimal and our objective was to learn as much as we could, when we could. It was unlikely that I would be placed in another situation where I would be able to witness a birth, assist in surgery, share an elderly patient's final moments, stitch, prod and poke people of all ages, all within weeks of each other. I felt like the children's TV character Mr Benn with the many and varied adventures he went on, although instead of a black bowler hat, I had a pink stethoscope.

I was well aware of the academic disadvantages that came with dyslexia and dyscalculia. I needed to work twice as hard as my peers to get at least average exam results, so I made the executive decision to start my revision for end-of-year exams more or less straight after the course began. Of course, I had to get a few lectures under my belt first in order to actually have something to learn and revise, but I was pretty much revising for exams from start to finish.

Nothing much went into my memory during the lectures themselves, unless there was a condition-specific patient anecdote shared by the lecturer that I found funny or particularly fascinating. Other than that, it was very much a case of in one ear and out the other, despite my best efforts. Generally, there were terms and phrases that I highlighted on my printed handout, which I would scribble notes on ferociously within the lecture. However, most of my learning happened outside of the classroom. Armed with my two-tone blue glasses, multicoloured revision cards, highlighters, blue pens, and everything else that my undergraduate course had taught me my dyslexic brain needed, I would head home or to the library after the day's lectures to translate them into information that I could remember.

In the first year, after informing the university about my SpLD diagnosis, I was given a needs assessment to work out the support I would require for the remainder of the physician associate course. I felt that I needed less support than I'd received as an undergraduate because I had already learned a lot of skills that I could apply again. From what was offered, I decided that the most useful options were extra time in the written exams to accommodate my slower reading and writing speed, and a room to myself so that I could read aloud without disturbing the rest of my classmates. They would be under enough stress and pressure without having to listen to me mumble to myself for hours and hours.

In both years, our end-of-year exams were in two formats, mirroring the two main ways of teaching on the course. The written exam was made up of single best answer (SBA) questions, requiring us to demonstrate a lot of our knowledge from our lecture-based learning. I had never taken an SBA examination before and immediately likened it to a light-hearted multiple-choice quiz – the kind where if you don't know the answer, you can guess and, thanks to chance and probability, some answers will inevitably be right.

However, whilst guesswork could perhaps work in our favour with a couple of questions, the exam paper was much harder than I'd originally thought. The emphasis was on the single *best* answer, not the single *correct* answer.

Often, more than one of the answers were right, but one of them was the best and we only gained the mark for selecting this option.

The other way in which we were tested was through an objective structured clinical examination (OSCE), consisting of roleplay scenarios using actors, and incorporating a lot of the clinical and communication skills we'd learned and practised on our placements. We sat this exam in a ward-like environment with a clinical bed, each small cubicle area curtained off from the others. Inside the cubicle would be an actor pretending to be a patient and an examiner marking how well we worked through the scenario explained on a piece of paper given to us in each station.

I hadn't told many of my classmates about my SpLD. There were some with whom I had a closer relationship than others, so I felt comfortable to share it with them, and other times, it was relevant to mention it, but generally it wasn't something that I broadcast. However, I hadn't considered the implications of not sharing this information widely when our first written exam came around.

As requested, I was given a private room to sit my written exam, meaning that I was missing from the main examination room where my peers were. After I had finished my written paper and my exam invigilator had taken it away, I turned my phone back on and was flooded with messages from concerned classmates, wondering where I had been for the exam. Some were worried that I had overslept, was unwell or had been hit by a bus on my walk into university.

Their concern, whilst touching, filled me with guilt that I had been on their mind during their exam. The next time that we were all together, I made sure to explain that I would take my written exams in a separate room and have extra time. I didn't go into details as to why, but they would have had a good idea. And for the rest of the written exams on the course, they wouldn't have to worry about my whereabouts.

Whilst having to complete two very different examinations was twice as stressful as just preparing for one, I appreciated there was a variety of knowledge and skills required to be a physician associate. A student could have memorised the entire medications book known as the *BNF* and all of the clinical textbooks in print, but without the communication skills required to speak to patients, they wouldn't be a good physician associate. Similarly, they could capture the magical skill of talking to patients, immediately making them feel cared for and comfortable under the student's care, but if they didn't have the clinical knowledge, they also wouldn't make a good physician associate. The profession requires high standards in both clinical knowledge and practical and communication skills, and our examinations helped us remember and prepare for this.

I would describe myself generally as a people person. A

confident introvert, with high levels of empathy and the ability to talk to strangers with ease. So on clinical placements, what I lacked in knowledge (before reading up on my learnings when I got home), I made up for in enabling patients to feel comfortable and at ease. I took full advantage of my time on clinical placements, talking and practising communication with patients at every opportunity I was given.

My clinical knowledge was a different story. The pathophysiology of disease and human anatomy, particularly all the names of the bones, was something that I struggled to learn, but I constantly made myself aware of the gaps in my knowledge, always keen to fill them.

One of our lecturers liked to tell us, 'It isn't required of you to know everything, but to be aware of what you don't know.' Unfortunately for me – and perhaps it's the same for all clinicians – the more I knew, the more I realised I didn't know. This turned into a constant quest to stay up to date with medical knowledge, guidelines and clinical advances that seemed to change more frequently than I would have preferred.

In preparing for my written SBA exam at the end of the second year, I revised until the words on the page had lost all meaning. I went to my allocated room where my invigilator was waiting for me, and where it felt like I'd already spent an eternity. Initially, I felt a little sorry for her having to take hours and hours out of her day to sit in a room and listen to me talk to myself, but the more I thought about it, the more I realised that being given the opportunity to sit quietly, reading a book of my choice and getting paid for the pleasure, wasn't something that I would have minded.

I stayed in my exam room until my time was up, even though we were allowed to leave once we felt we had finished the paper. One booklet contained the questions, and another sheet was where we shaded in the circular box corresponding to the right answer. I remember the course director repeatedly telling us not to put our answers into the question booklet itself, but only on the answer sheet as this was specially formatted to be put into a machine, which would grade our papers automatically through being able to identify the answer we had selected.

Missing out on the opportunity to glance at my peers and see what they were doing as I filled in my own answer sheet made me worry that I might still do the wrong thing, despite repeatedly being told the correct method. Interestingly, although I was alone with no-one else to corroborate what I was doing, it wasn't I but a couple of my peers in the room with everyone else who made the mistake of putting their answers on the wrong sheet. Their answers were still collected and graded, but by hand, likely to the marker's mild annoyance.

The wait for the exam results was standard – agonisingly long and unkind. It reminded me of GCSE and A-level results, where we'd been expected to wait patiently for months and months to find out our fate. The best thing I could do was put the results out of my mind entirely, or I could have ended up spending the entire summer worrying about something I no longer had any control over and couldn't change.

When the overall final exam results were due to be released, I remember being glued to whichever electronic device I had to hand at the time, whether phone or laptop, with my university email inbox open, regularly refreshing the page. When the email came through after hours of clicking and refreshing, I couldn't open it fast enough.

I was devastated, embarrassed and downhearted to learn that I had failed my final exams. I had failed both the written SBA paper and the roleplaying OSCE. The déjà vu was awful as I thought back to the end of my first year on the physician associate course, where I had also failed both of my exams. After having spent the summer holiday studying hard and revising like there was no tomorrow, I had been able to pass the first-year resit exams, enabling me to continue into the second year with the rest of my classmates.

I had thought that I'd cracked the code and found the way to get through my second year exams, but was sadly mistaken and found myself riding the same rollercoaster of emotions as a year ago, including disappointment, envy at my classmates who'd passed, and general sadness. I felt like I had worked harder than anyone else on the course, having started revising for this exam right at the beginning, but I knew ultimately it wasn't about working hard, it was about working smart.

It was some consolation to know that, just like with my first-year exams, I wasn't the only person on the course who didn't pass. Some consolation, but not much.

The second year exams were familiar to us all, with the same format and similar medical questions and scenarios as the first year, but they were slightly harder and there was much more pressure as a lot was riding on them. The exam results for the second year also determined whether we were able to go on to pass the national exams, ultimately determining whether would pass the entire course and become qualified physician associates, or not.

The university's halls of residence, where I still lived, were quiet as the rest of the students had moved out and gone back home for the summer, which helped reduce my distractions. I was still working as an RA once a week, but at this point, the phone I had to respond to was hardly ever ringing.

For both years of the course, the university held its own exams, and then the national exams followed. It was compulsory to pass both. The national exams followed the same structure as the SBA and OSCE, but were standardised, meaning that everyone, regardless of which university they were at, sat the same paper. This made sure that physician associate students from both St George's and Aberdeen were examined fairly and in the same way.

The University OSCE examinations had about 12 stations and we would move through them one by one, eventually completing the whole circuit. We were given a couple of minutes before each scenario started, to read the information card, providing us with all the relevant details for the station. Then we were timed to carry out the scenario, referring back to the card whenever we needed to. The scenarios were all procedures we had done many, many times whilst practising with each other and on placement with real patients. The difference this time was that our patient was an actor, and we were being assessed in everything that we did and said.

For the second year OSCE examinations, the university hired professional actors to play our patients. In one of the stations, my 'patient' was an actress I recognised from *EastEnders*. This actress had had a particularly sad storyline in the soap and I had felt sorry for her ever since. The hardest thing for me in that moment was to see her as the patient as briefed on my card and not the *EastEnders* character. I think it worked well. And she was a great actress, embracing her ailment in true form.

Through sweat, many tears and lots of prayer, I passed the second year University resit exams allowing me to go on to sit the national exams with the rest of my peers, which I passed. Finally, I was able to call myself a fully qualified physician associate.

Career day was something that I had been looking forward to. Timetabled towards the end of our second year on the course, before our final exams, it was a day away from the placement rotations and the classroom, and was like an oasis in the middle of the desert.

Career day was where potential employers were invited to talk to us about vacancies they had or were soon to have in their wards, clinics and departments. The physician associate profession was new and exciting at the time, and everyone wanted to have one on their clinical team. It was also an opportunity for potential employers to ask us questions about our career choice, and for us to ask them about their specialties.

The potential employers came from all across the UK, from both primary and secondary care, and were all given an opportunity to pitch themselves to us. It was a day where I not only didn't need to either retain or regurgitate medical knowledge or clinical management skills, but also, along with my classmates, felt extremely valuable and wanted, and that felt great.

Being a physician associate can sometimes be bittersweet. On clinical placement, there were members of staff who seemed excited about the new role and the extra medical support that we would be able to offer. There were others, though, who were less positive, some believing that we would be stepping on doctors' toes, and some who felt that we might be unsafe around patients, having done a much shorter course than our doctor colleagues. The thing was, we were not training or trying to be doctors; we were physician associates, a completely different role and scope of practice. And now, we were all keen to show just what we could do.

Each potential employer would deliver a small talk or PowerPoint presentation to us, outlining what working as a physician associate in their department would look like, the benefits and why we should join them. It reminded me of an inverted version of the popular TV show *Dragons' Den* with the employers pitching to us, the investment that they were seeking in the form not of cash, but our skills.

By this time, some of the people on my course already had jobs lined up. In fact, one of my colleagues had been offered a job after qualification a whole nine months before we even took our final university and national exams. Some didn't have jobs, but knew exactly what specialty they wanted to work in, and some just wanted a chance to sleep in, watch films and not think about medicine at all for a little while after the course had finished.

I was in the last group, but I had chosen my specialty, so was also keeping my eyes and ears open for amazing general practice opportunities. At the time, a part of me felt a little jealous that some of my colleagues would walk straight into a job as soon as they received their pass mark. On the other hand, whilst sitting and listening to the potential employers outlining all the opportunities and trying to persuade us to join them, I liked not yet having any commitments and being able to keep an open mind.

One reason I liked this was that it reduced the pressure. I couldn't imagine having an employer wait nine months for me to start the job. In that time, they would surely have built up in their head an image of what they assumed a physician associate would be able to do and bring to the department, with all the potential that held for them to be disappointed when I started. Another plus to not having committed to a physician associate post was that it left me open to hearing about new jobs and opportunities that I might never have considered.

I listened attentively to the hospital specialty pitches, but felt sure that there was nothing those potential employers could say that would make me prefer their setting to general practice. I had done enough clinical placements to know that the hospital wasn't where my passion lay and I had eyes for general practice alone.

There was a variety of people pitching GP opportunities. Some were from large practices, others small. Some were local to the area, others further out. But the presentation that stood out to me came from a GP practice partner who had prepared a presentation that spoke fondly of the staff, the patients and, last but not least, Maisie the practice dog. Despite being a large practice, it was portrayed as having a friendly, warm team, where staff were open and excited about the new skills their very first physician associate could bring.

After the presentations, we were given opportunities to mingle with the speakers over tea, coffee and biscuits. Naturally, I made a beeline for the practice partner who had piqued my interest. I wondered whether an informal chat about his practice would leave me as interested as his presentation had done.

A couple of other classmates had gathered around him

and were asking him questions, but I knew deep down that this practice was where I wanted to go. At the end of the session, we were given a sheet of paper with the details and email addresses of all the speakers in attendance. I contacted the GP practice the same evening and asked to visit and have a look around.

There was another GP practice that I contacted to ask for an informal visit after hearing its representative's presentation at our career day. Whilst I was much less interested in this practice, I thought it would be good to see and speak to more than one potential employer. This practice, about a mile away from the one that I was really interested in, invited me in for an informal visit and chat, as I had hoped.

The train journey to the practice was very straightforward, but once I got off the train, Google Maps couldn't decide which direction I should be walking in. I had given myself plenty of time to find the practice, aware of my difficulties, but on this warm summer afternoon, the extra time seemed to disappear rather rapidly, leaving me only a few minutes to get on to the right path.

The problem I'd found was that the map was telling me to walk along a busy main road, which didn't seem right. What I hadn't realised was that there was a well-trodden grass footpath running adjacent to the road. I didn't see it until a fellow pedestrian casually strolled along it with her large black dog.

Eventually, after walking along the well-hidden path, dangerously close to cars whizzing by, circumnavigating a large pond twice whilst trying to be obedient to my phone's confusing directions, asking two different strangers for help, I found where I needed to be. Despite having called ahead to apologise about my lateness, I was embarrassed and just wanted to go home and cry into my pillow. The practice manager assured me that it wasn't a problem and said the partners were waiting for me. This surprised me as I had been expecting to have a chat with just one of the GP partners, not all of them.

After leading me along a corridor, the practice manager opened a large, heavy wooden door and invited me to go into the room. There, I was met by a group of friendly but slightly warm and flustered GP partners, sitting around a brown oak table.

This was an interview.

I had asked to have a look around their practice, nothing more, and here I was, 30 minutes late for my own interview. They were friendly and kind before I'd even explained that I had got lost, but despite their forgiving ways, I couldn't shake the feeling that I had ruined everything and didn't shine as brightly in the surprise interview as I usually would have.

I wasn't offered the post, but took many lessons from the experience. I needed to give myself way more time to follow directions. I would much rather arrive far too early and kill time reading my fully charged Kindle, which lived in my bag, desperate to be read after two years of neglect whilst I was on the course. I also decided always to have a few prepared responses to typical interview questions in my back pocket, just in case another informal conversation turned out to be a surprise interview. I had heard of physician associates being interviewed while walking along a corridor, then offered a job on the spot. That was never going to happen to me if the pressure of being caught out made me even forget my own last name.

Luckily, this all happened well before my interview at the practice that I really wanted to go to. A few months passed between the GP partner coming to the university to speak at the career day, and the practice putting out its physician associate vacancy, but I had stopped looking at other opportunities, patiently waiting for the advert to be placed so that I could apply.

After a couple of months of waiting, I emailed the practice manager, asking if they were still looking to hire a physician associate. They were indeed, but were first sorting out a few things. The following week, the advert was put out and I applied immediately.

I was invited in for an interview and was a little surprised to see some familiar faces in the practice waiting room as we waited to be called in for our turn. A couple of my classmates had also applied for the post, but I tried not to let the competition put me off. All I could do was my best. I had become used to my colleagues passing exams that I had failed and excelling where I didn't, but despite the initial knocks in confidence, this really did help my resilience. If this job was the one for me, I would get it, and if I was unsuccessful, there would be an even better job waiting for me.

The interview went well. The GPs were so friendly, I had to remind myself that they were total strangers. From the ease of the conversation, you would have thought we had known each other for years.

I was offered the job that I wanted and had waited for so patiently. My friend had been offered a job at the practice where I had flunked my surprise interview, which was where she really wanted to work. So we both ended up exactly where we wanted to be.

Because my practice had delayed placing its advert, I'd had some time after completing the course to finally have a breather and a rest. This was another benefit of not having a job waiting for me: I could just enjoy the gift of free time. I could watch TV in the evenings without guilt. I could go to sleep and wake up whenever my body decided. I could read books for pleasure again, and not just for my academic learning. I could go into central London and walk around aimlessly being a tourist, something I hadn't really had much time to do before now, despite living in the city for two years.

I rationalised that there wasn't much point in starting a brand-new career tired and exhausted. Plus with all the resit examinations I'd had to do, I had earned my rest. I needed time to regroup, refocus, and then get ready to start again, but this time wearing a different hat to the student one I had become so used to.

As graduation for the course happened quite late in the calendar year, a new term had started at the university during this time. After discussion with my boss, I was able to continue working as an RA for a few more months, as until graduation, I was still technically a postgraduate student, and thereby qualified for the role. I continued to live at the university halls of residence while I looked for somewhere more appropriate to move to next.

I was able to start running again, freely, unbothered by how slowly or how long I was hitting the pavement. On one of my runs, I decided to go past the GP practice, just to see it, as it was only three miles away from the university halls of residence. Once I reached my destination, I sat on the wall across the road, looking up at the large four storey building that I would soon call my workplace, reflective and grateful, as well as sweaty and breathless. After waiting for my breathing to return to normal, I decided to walk back home, taking in the unfamiliar area as I did so.

I hadn't been the smartest, quickest or most confident physician associate on my course, but I still knew that I was a great physician associate. I had learned, grown, persevered and blossomed, and was ready to put every experience so far into good practice. The differences in how I understand, interpret and get through day-to-day life, now known to be part of SpLD, are all things that have helped make me who I am, and the diagnosis hadn't taken any of that away; it had just given me context.

A few weeks later, I started my new job. In my clinical room with my very own name plaque on the door, I called my first patient in via the automated screen that flashed their name in the waiting room. Then I stood in the doorway to beckon to the patient if they forgot where they needed to go. The corridor was long and my room was right at the end, which was to result in patients often forgetting my room number before they were even halfway.

A young female approached. She saw the number on my door and smiled as I stood aside to allow her into the room.

'Good morning, I'm Chloe, and I'm the physician associate. How can I help you today?'

Epilogue

Statutory regulation of the physician associate profession is something that I – and my colleagues – have been hoping and waiting for since before I joined the course, and we are still waiting many years later. In the meantime, the Faculty of Physician Associates at the Royal College of Physicians has a managed voluntary register which all physician associates are strongly encouraged to join. Most employers won't even consider a physician associate for employment without them being on this register.

The register provides assurance that the physician associate has qualified from an appropriate UK or US programme, has passed national examinations and mandatory recertification exams every six years*, has continuing professional development of a minimum of 50 hours per year, which includes things like training courses, and doesn't have any code of conduct, scope of practice or fitness to practice concerns. Statutory regulation, however, would provide physician associates the opportunity to be fully embedded and recognised within the NHS across both primary and secondary care, helping to shape health-care and continually contribute to the needs of the patient, delivering high-quality care.

Physician associates are not doctors. We do not pretend to be doctors and are forthcoming about our title, limitations of skill and knowledge. We are dependent prac-titioners who are able to make independent decisions and work clinically with the supervision of a named senior doctor, who remains on hand to discuss clinical cases, give advice and review the patient, if necessary, enabled by collaborative and supportive working relationships. Physi-cian associates cannot prescribe medication or request ionising radiations like X-rays or CT scans, but we are able to increase clinical capacity, never replacing, but supporting doctors and those working within the clinical team.

The good feeling that I had about my practice after listening to the GP partner deliver his presentation on the morning of the career day was definitely accurate, as I have stayed and remained employed there for the past ten years. The GP partner has since moved on to pastures new, as has Maisie the dog, but the essence of the practice remains the same and I still enjoy working there, even after all this time.

After starting as the practice's first ever physician associate, I was a team of one for a few years. I now belong to a team of four, working alongside my wonderful physician associate colleagues each day. There have been changes in staffing, ways of working and a whole global pandemic during my time at the practice. But even so, I wouldn't change my decision to be a physician associate, and hope that those uncertain about the profession will realise how great it really is.

*The process of physician associate revalidation has recently changed. Instead of the 6 yearly recertification exams, it is now instead compulsory for physician associates to evidence continuing professional development (CPD) as per the FPA guidance until such time as the GMC regulation and revalidation come in.

References

Riedel, S (2005) 'Edward and the history of smallpox and vaccination' *National Library of Medicine* 18 (1) 21-25 Available at https://www.ncbi.nlm.nih.gov/pmc/articles/PMC1200696/ Last Accessed 10/02/2024

Acknowledgments

Writing a book is a journey that navigates solitary paths but is never a solo endeavour. I am deeply grateful to the individuals and resources who have been instrumental in bringing this work to fruition.

First and foremost, I offer heartfelt thanks to God for being the source of creativity, inspiration, purpose, and resilience in this literary endeavour. This work is a testament to His blessings and grace.

BIG LOVE to my family for their unwavering support and understanding during the countless hours spent lost in the world of words. Your patience and encouragement has been my guiding light. Mum and Dad (Karen and Mark), Josh, Jacob, Nanny Viv, and Aunty Nikki, my superstars. Grandad Sheppey, Nanny Beryl and Nanny Bertha, I'm sorry that you weren't able to read this, but I think it would have made you proud.

To my friends, Putneymead colleagues past and present, and church family, thank you for your encouragement, constructive feedback, and the occasional nudge to keep going when the writing process seemed too daunting. Beverley, Benjamina, Katrina, Katherine, Nikki, Natasha, Melisa, Jemima, Joan and Dan my cheerleaders. Bookclub babes Michelle and Frances, you are amazing. Jeannie and Karen, thank you for your help, encouragement, contributions and kind quotes for this book. Alex and Martin, thank you for everything.

To my St George's Physician Associate studies cohort (2012-2014), what a ride! It was a pleasure to study with you all.

Sue Lascelles my writing mentor, your dedication to the craft has been empowering. Alison Jack my editor who whose keen insights and meticulous attention to detail have helped shape this book into its final form. Emma Ewbank, a heartfelt thank you for not only crafting the beautiful book cover and materials that encapsulates the essence of my story, but also for your creativity, direction and kindness.

Lastly, to my readers, thank you so much for your interest, curiosity, kindness, support and reviews. I hope that my book provides you with inspiration, hope and clinical wonder.

ABOUT THE AUTHOR

Chloe is a writer and Physician Associate and *Good Practice: Confessions of a physician associate student* is her debut memoir. You can find out more about Chloe on her website at www.chloebrathwaite.co.uk, where you can also subscribe to her newsletter.

If you enjoyed this book, please leave a review on Amazon and/ or Goodreads. Each review is greatly appreciated and helps to find more readers who may enjoy this book too.